T0215348

# Hermeneutic Phenomenology in Health and Social Care Research

This book explores how, why and when hermeneutic phenomenology can be used as a methodology in health and social research.

Providing actual examples of doing robust hermeneutic phenomenology and a focus on praxis, the book demonstrates how philosophical or theoretical notions can inform, enrich and enhance our research projects. The chapters offer examples of many different research designs and interpretive decisions in order to illustrate the unbounded and creative nature of this type of inquiry, whilst also demonstrating the trustworthiness of the scientific processes adopted. The chapter authors invite the reader on a unique journey that highlights how they made individual and tailored decisions throughout their projects, emphasising the challenges and joys they encountered.

This book is a valuable resource for all students and academics who wish to explore the meaningfulness of human lived experiences across the multitude of phenomena in health and social care.

**Susan Crowther** is a Professor of midwifery at Auckland University of Technology in Aotearoa, New Zealand. Her research interests are mainly focused on midwifery, maternity and women's health, although she explores myriad topics with postgraduate students from a variety of disciplines/professions. She has published two books: "Joy at birth" (sole author), "Spirituality and Childbirth" with co-editor Dr. Jenny Hall and another book coming in 2022: "Mindfulness across the childbirth sphere" with co-editor Dr. Lorna Davies. Susan is a member of three editorial boards, sits on review panels and enjoys supervising postgraduate degrees. Contacts/links: E. susan.crowther@aut.ac.nz – Twitter: @SusanCrowtherMW – Blog/webpage: https://drsusancrowther.com/.

**Gill Thomson** is a Professor in Perinatal Health at the University of Central Lancashire in North-West, U.K. Gill's research interests centre around perinatal health and wellbeing and lay/peer support models of care. Gill's used hermeneutic phenomenology in her Ph.D., she supervises Ph.D. students using this approach, and she co-facilitates the annual hermeneutic phenomenology methodology course with Susan. Gill has authored over 100 peer-reviewed publications and is the lead editor of two Routledge texts (*Qualitative research in childbirth* *and midwifery: Phenomenological approaches* (2011), and *Psychosocial resilience and risk in the perinatal period: Implications and guidance for professionals* (2017)). Gill is an editorial member of two journals and a steering group member of SCENE (SCENE | SCENE (utu.fi) – an international network dedicated to improving neonatal care. Contacts/links: Email – Gthomson@uclan.ac.uk; Twitter @gill_thomson; Webpage – Gill Thomson – UCLan.

# Hermeneutic Phenomenology in Health and Social Care Research

Edited by Susan Crowther
and Gill Thomson

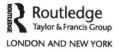
Routledge
Taylor & Francis Group

LONDON AND NEW YORK

First published 2023
by Routledge
4 Park Square, Milton Park, Abingdon, Oxon OX14 4RN

and by Routledge
605 Third Avenue, New York, NY 10158

*Routledge is an imprint of the Taylor & Francis Group, an informa business*

© 2023 selection and editorial matter, **Susan Crowther and Gill Thomson;** individual chapters, the contributors

*British Library Cataloguing-in-Publication Data*
A catalogue record for this book is available from the British Library

*Library of Congress Cataloging-in-Publication Data*
A catalog record has been requested for this book

ISBN: 978-0-367-53379-3 (hbk)
ISBN: 978-1-032-28582-5 (pbk)
ISBN: 978-1-003-08166-1 (ebk)

DOI: 10.4324/9781003081661

Typeset in Goudy
by KnowledgeWorks Global Ltd.

To all scholarship past, present and future that seeks to reveal what it means to be alive. To all our colleagues who came before who shared their wisdom and vision – we acknowledge we stand upon the shoulders of giants as we reach out for further understanding about the experience of being human. As we all walk our paths, we acknowledge that the way is decorated and illuminated by the lessons and teachings of the past; and as we think, write and encourage ourselves and others, we are reminded that we are the inspiration that we have been waiting for.

# Contents

# Figures

# Tables

# Contributors

**Lesley Dibley** is a Professor of Qualitative Nursing Research at The University of Greenwich, London, England. Her research interests are phenomenologically driven, including her Ph.D. on the experience of stigma in people with inflammatory bowel disease. She leads the Centre for Chronic Illness and Ageing in the Institute for Lifecourse Development at the University of Greenwich, and with Professor Suzanne Dickerson, Dr. Mel Duffy and Professor Annie Vandermause, co-authored the recent textbook entitled "Doing hermeneutic phenomenological research: a practical guide." L.B.Dibley@Greenwich.ac.uk

**Christine Sorrell Dinkins** is the Kenan Professor of Philosophy at Wofford College in South Carolina, U.S.A., where she teaches courses in Ancient Greek Philosophy, Phenomenological Research Methods and Philosophy of Medicine. She pioneered Socratic Shared Inquiry as a qualitative research method, a method used today in many dissertations in the social science and healthcare disciplines. Her current scholarship focuses on Socratic-hermeneutic phenomenological research with undergraduate collaborators seeking to amplify the voices of underserved and minoritised communities.

**Jean Duckworth** is a Senior Lecturer at the University of Central Lancashire. After training in law and then homeopathy, she practised as a homeopath and lecturer. This led to her undertaking a Ph.D. using Heideggerian hermeneutic phenomenology to explore the experience of midwife homeopaths. Jean is an active researcher and supervises doctoral students across a number of health disciplines. JEDuckworth@uclan.ac.uk

**Christine Edwards'** ongoing achievements stem from executive corporate HRM positions and a background in education, training and development. Christine is currently a lecturer in the post-graduate programs in the Business and Hospitality vertical at Torrens University Australia (TUA). Christine's research focus is Human Resource Management and Leadership. Christine's research interests lie in hermeneutic phenomenology: uncovering taken-for-granted understandings of the lived experience. christine.edwards@torrens.edu.au

**Helen F. Harrison** is a professor in the School of Nursing at Fanshawe College in London, Ontario, Canada. She teaches courses in "Holistic Health Assessment"

and "Anatomy & Physiology." Helen has practiced as a Registered Nurse and Nurse Practitioner in many settings including acute inpatient medicine, family planning and population-based research on hereditary hemochromatosis. She has a longstanding fascination with the human body, and her research interests include professional education, embodied knowing, hermeneutic phenomenology and student peer mentorship in higher education. hfharris@uwo.ca

**Lesley Kay** is an Associate Professor of Midwifery at City, University of London. Her research interests are centred on women's expectations and experiences of birth, particularly how birth stories might shape the way that women experience birth, spirituality and birth and global and respectful midwifery care. Lesley's interest and engagement with hermeneutic phenomenology was ignited when she attended the "Institute for Heideggerian Hermeneutical Methodologies" at Indiana University. Lesley is currently the Divisional Lead for Midwifery and Radiography at City, University of London and the Lead Midwife for Education. lesley.kay@city.ac.uk

**Elizabeth "Anne" Kinsella** is Professor and Director of the Institute of Health Sciences Education in the Faculty of Medicine and Health Sciences at McGill University in Montreal, Canada. Anne's interdisciplinary scholarship focuses on professional education, practice and policy in health and social care professions. She is particularly interested in reflective/reflexive practices, embodiment, phenomenologies of practice, phronesis and epistemic justice. Anne is a qualitative researcher and educational philosopher and teaches "Philosophical foundations of qualitative research." elizabeth.kinsella@mcgill. ca; Twitter @EaKinsella.

**Polly Livermore** is a part-time Matron at Great Ormond Street Children's Hospital and part-time NIHR GOSH BRC Clinical Academic lead for nurses and allied health professionals. In this latter role, Polly spends time supporting masters, Ph.D. and postdoctoral students to advance their research skills, specifically in qualitative research and phenomenology. Her NIHR clinical doctoral research fellowship used Heideggerian hermeneutic phenomenology to explore the experiences of children and young people with Juvenile Dermatomyositis. Polly is the lead Paediatric Rheumatology nurse for the United Kingdom and is an Associate Editor of Rheumatology Advances in Practice. polly.livermore@ucl.ac.uk

**Kent Smith** is a counsellor in private practice who uses phenomenology as a philosophy towards caring and helping others. It was lucky he found that Heideggerian phenomenology just happens to be a philosophy that you can use as a research methodology, from there, everything has changed. His experience of completing a doctorate, which revealed the notion of "leaderful," drew him back into his counselling practice in a new and wonderful way. kentsmith. research@gmail.com

**Liz Smythe** is an Emeritus Professor in the process of retiring from the Auckland University of Technology. She was first a nurse and then moved on to midwifery.

Her Ph.D. was her grounding in Heideggerian hermeneutic phenomenology. Since then, she has supervised many masters and doctoral students as they too explored lived experience. She has worked closely with Deb Spence over many years. liz.smythe@aut.ac.nz

**Margot Solomon** retired from the department of psychotherapy at Auckland University of Technology in Aotearoa, New Zealand, in 2020. Her doctorate, using Heideggerian hermeneutic phenomenology, was a later in life endeavour, and was a way of reflecting on many years of teaching. It helped her to see what she knew but did not know she knew. She now works in private practice as a group-analytic and psychoanalytic psychotherapist. margotps@mac.com

**Deb Spence** is a Senior Lecturer in the throes of retiring from Auckland University of Technology. Primarily a nurse but also a midwife, her Ph.D. drew from Gadamer to articulate the experience of nursing people from cultures other than one's own. She has supervised students from a range of health disciplines who have undertaken qualitative research mostly from a hermeneutic phenomenological perspective. deb.spence@aut.ac.nz

**Joshua Spier** is an experienced community development practitioner, qualitative researcher and social planner with a focus on disability access and inclusion, public health planning and monitoring community wellbeing. Recent achievements include development, oversight and implementation of high-level organisational plans that respond to changing community needs, government policy and legislative requirements – committed to participatory social planning and facilitating partnerships for community wellbeing outcomes. In 2018 published the monograph from his doctoral work Heidegger and the Lived Experience of Being a University Educator. joshuaspier@gmail.com

**Bridget Taylor** spent her working career on parallel yet complementary paths: she was a senior specialist nurse in community palliative care as well as a senior lecturer at Oxford Brookes University. Her Ph.D. provided the opportunity to combine her two areas of speciality: palliative care and sexuality and intimacy. It also established her grounding in hermeneutic phenomenology. She has recently retired though she maintains an active role in supporting hermeneutic researchers. bridgettaylor1@gmail.com

# Foreword

Appearance necessarily occurs in some light. Only by virtue of light ... can what shines show itself, that is, radiate. But brightness in its turn rests upon something open, something free, which might illuminate it.

Martin Heidegger, "The End of Philosophy
and the Task of Thinking" (1969/1993, 383)

The book you are holding in your hands is a bringer of light, of freedom to explore, of the openness required for phenomenological engagement with the world and ourselves. It may look like a heavy tome to those less familiar with hermeneutic phenomenology research, but I assure you, it is light, or rather it is luminous. For any reader, a delve into the chapters of this book will yield a rare opportunity to see the rich variety of methods, approaches and attitudes that phenomenological research not only can include but must include. The editors of this anthology and the authors of each chapter let you in to see the *how* and *why* of their research, to show to all researchers from novice to expert that there are not just one or two or even 100 "right" ways to do phenomenology. Phenomenology is done "right" when the researcher remains open and allows the phenomenon to reveal itself.

I will begin by introducing myself. I am a philosopher who works with nurses who work with philosophy. My scholarship is at the intersection of Plato and Heidegger, combining Socratic method and hermeneutic phenomenology. My mother is a nurse educator and researcher, and in collaboration with her, I discovered a beautiful world of health and social care scholars who adopt the theories of Husserl, Heidegger, Gadamer, Arendt, Merleau-Ponty, Stein and others to inform their approach to studying lived experience.

Many years ago, when I was an undergraduate, I took a Heidegger seminar, and my life and my thinking have not been the same since. As I now tell my own undergraduate students, "After about 5 or 6 weeks of studying phenomenology, a light will come on for you, a switch will flip. And once the switch flips and you see the world with a phenomenological mindset, you can't go back." When I say this to my students, it is both a warning and a promise. To engage with phenomenological theories and research is to see the world anew, to see the unseen, to become a combination of ally and bystander and agent in allowing hidden things to come into the light. I truly believe that to teach someone to see the world with a phenomenological mindset is a gift that will stay with them their whole lives.

If one wishes to see things phenomenologically, to *research* phenomena in this way, one can study the theories and the variety of recommended methods, but in the end, each study is unique, involving its own journey for the researcher and the participants. That uniqueness of each journey is the biggest reason I am excited for this book to join the world of scholarship on hermeneutic phenomenology. Instead of a how-to, it's a "we'll show you," a glimpse behind the curtain that lets us see how experienced, respected researchers find their own new way with each phenomenon they study.

Gadamer maintains that "*what constitutes the essence of research is much less merely applying the usual methods than discovering new ones – and underlying that, the creative imagination of the scientist*" (1960/1989, 551–552). In this anthology, we get to see researchers discovering those new methods or inventing them as they go along; we get to read about studies with widely diverse phenomena and ways of attuning to those phenomena.

As Socrates says in Plato's *Euthyphro*, "*The lover of inquiry must follow his beloved*" (1981, 14b). Quite similarly, Heidegger in *Being and Time* states, "*As a seeking, questioning needs previous guidance from what it seeks*" (1927/1993, 45). The phenomenon itself must guide our inquiry, and thus the most experienced researcher should still be adapting and experimenting with methodology with each new phenomenon they study.

In Plato's famous cave allegory, we find prisoners chained in a cave since birth, not knowing their cave is only a cave, mistaking the cave for the real world. When a prisoner escapes and sees the sun and the world as it truly is, he tries to go back into the cave to tell the others, but they cannot understand him and dismiss his claims as gibberish. The point, Socrates says at the end of his story, is that we cannot put understanding directly into a soul by simply stating the truth or handing out knowledge. Instead, we must guide and support others on their path out of the cave. We must "*turn the whole body toward the light*" (Plato, 1992, 518c). In the original context, Socrates is speaking about the path to moral enlightenment, but I believe the same sort of journey is necessary to reach phenomenological understanding and attunement. To go from seeing the world filtered through our own assumptions and determinations to allowing the phenomena of the world to un-conceal themselves as we safeguard their truth – that is just as difficult and as rewarding a journey.

A mutually supporting journey up to the light of phenomenological understanding is what this book has to offer all of us. For more novice readers, it may be a journey out of the darkness of confusion or frustration. For more expert readers, it may be a nudge to experiment or a refreshing shake-up of approaches they have grown too comfortable with. For all readers, it will be a journey of discovery. Whether you are a teacher or student, an expert or novice, I encourage you to read these chapters with an open heart as well as mind, to join these researchers as they reflect on their own research journeys. And may all of us, as a community of researchers, collaborate and learn from one another so that we may always walk together up into the light.

*Christine Sorrell Dinkins*
*Spartanburg, South Carolina, U.S.A.*
*December 2021*

## References

Gadamer, H. 1960/1989. *Truth and Method* (2nd revised ed.). Trans. J. Weinsheimer and D. G. Marshall. New York: Continuum.

Heidegger, M. 1927/1993. "Being and Time: Introduction." *Basic Writings.* D. Krell, Ed. (Trans. J. Stambaugh). New York, NY: Harper Collins.

Heidegger, M. 1969/1993. "The End of Philosophy and the Task of Thinking." *Basic Writings.* D. Krell, Ed. (Trans. J. Stambaugh). New York, NY: Harper Collins.

Plato (trans. 1981). *Euthyphro.* Five Dialogues. Trans. G. M. A. Grube. Indianapolis, IN: Hackett.

Plato (trans. 1992). *Republic.* Trans. G. M. A. Grube and C. D. C. Reeve. Indianapolis, IN: Hackett.

# Acknowledgements

Thank you to all our authors – for your wonderful contributions and patience as you helped us achieve our vision. Also, a special mention to the most phenomenological individual we know – Professor Liz Smythe – your encouragement, generous spirit and belief have continued to be a special source of inspiration.

# 1 Introduction

## Situating hermeneutic phenomenology as research method in health, social care and education

*Susan Crowther and Gill Thomson*

### Preface

Welcome to this collection of chapters which we are thrilled to share with you all. Many of you would have come to this book new to the hermeneutic phenomenology philosophical orientation and seek understanding on how to apply this way of thinking to your research projects. You may be feeling hesitant about finding "the right way" to use the philosophical underpinnings as a methodology; some of you may be more seasoned and want further learning and perspectives. Some of you reading may have come to this book because you are supervising a postgraduate research student using this methodology and have not applied this approach before. Some of you may be asked to examine a hermeneutic phenomenology study or be part of a larger study that incorporates this approach. Whatever reason you have arrived today to this reading – welcome.

> Every questioning is a seeking. Every seeking takes its direction beforehand from what is sought. Questioning is a knowing search for beings in their thatness and whatness.
>
> Martin Heidegger, *Being and Time* (1995, 5)

### Genesis of an idea

Why this book? We (Susan and Gill) both have completed several hermeneutic phenomenological studies including our own doctoral research projects. We both supervise postgraduate students using hermeneutic phenomenological approaches and we have been delivering an international hermeneutic phenomenology course and symposium since 2016 in online and in-person formats. What has struck us both repeatedly are the challenges and anxiety of venturing into interpretive leaps necessary to bring forth an ontological depth to the inquiry that is the hallmark of great phenomenological reporting. We have witnessed how participants seem to struggle and flounder remaining unsure about how the road to completion will look. Friend and mentor, Professor Liz Smythe, offers the reassurance of "trust the process" – meaning that the depth of interpretation will come. However, this may not come easily for everyone. Trusting the process involves listening and being constantly reminded to let the data (e.g. interviews), or as Gadamer would say, the gathered understanding that opens a way to illuminating the phenomenon.

DOI: 10.4324/9781003081661-1

The hermeneutic phenomenological approach is increasingly used in health, educational and social science studies to collect and analyse lived experiential descriptions of a phenomenon. However, currently, there is a lack of guidance as to how to undertake these projects and, in particular, the use of philosophical concepts to guide methodological and interpretive decisions. Although there is literature and books detailing aspects and processes of doing hermeneutic phenomenology as an applied research project (e.g. Crist and Tanner 2003; Dibley et al. 2020; Smythe 2011; Thomson et al. 2011; van Manen 2014; Wilcke 2002), there is only some methodological guidance using actual in-depth examples; specifically, on the interpretive leaps required. We saw the need for a book that was concerned with praxis to offer in-depth insights to the hermeneutic phenomenological interpretive leap. This book addresses this need and brings together a gathering of authors from around the world with diverse backgrounds and interests.

Our purpose in this anthology is to show you how it is possible to find your way in taking those all-important interpretive leaps. Each author reveals how they learnt to "trust the process" and bring to their writing and thinking an idiosyncratic mood and inspiration. They invite you into their world and how they journeyed through their unique hermeneutic phenomenological journeys from the inception of the ideas through to how they reported the final interpretive analysis.

We acknowledge and appreciate there are challenges to doing hermeneutic phenomenology, such as having to complete this work within restrictive academic milestones of time constraints and wordage limitations. This can result in hasty interpretive findings and insufficient depth of scholarly writing over time that is required to communicate detailed transparent interpretive processes. This lack of detail, and, at times, congruence, has led to several attempts to discredit the credibility of this research approach (Paley 2016). This book arose as a response to these concerns and the desire to provide a comprehensive resource that would provide readers with actual "lived-through" examples of doing robust hermeneutic phenomenology focusing on *how* philosophical or theoretical notions can inform, enrich, transform, deepen, and enhance projects. In this book, we focus on praxis,[1] the chapter authors "show" and not "tell" how they achieve this.

## Situating co-editors

To be congruent with hermeneutic phenomenology, we draw on ourselves in a reflexive way. Throughout this chapter, as will be reflected in each chapter, we show how researchers need to come to this genre of research from a reflexive perspective that engages in an ongoing critical dialogue on human experiences. This helps illuminate our own pre-understandings and motivations for undertaking a study and the myriad directions our thinking can take us, and the many ways hermeneutic phenomenology can be enacted. In hermeneutic phenomenological studies, the methods and research processes are always written from a first-person perspective. To speak in the third person would be an anathema to the hermeneutic phenomenological enterprise and belie the ontological positioning of this form of scholarship. We are inviting you into our lives as researchers and people within contexts – to do otherwise would make little sense, and therefore you will note that throughout this book, personal pronouns are adopted, for example, my, I, we, our and you.

I (Susan) have been in healthcare since the early 80s and from the early 90s, midwifery. Born in the United Kingdom, I have worked and practiced across many global regions and had the honour to be at the birth of hundreds of births in every conceivable place. Although I have been out of clinical midwifery practice for some years – after being swallowed up into academia, I still identify myself as a midwife. I am married and have lived in Aotearoa, New Zealand, since 2006 with my Kiwi husband Toby and dog Flo. We live on a lifestyle block north of Auckland. After a stint in Aberdeen, Scotland, as a Professor of Midwifery (2015–2019), I returned to Auckland University of Technology (AUT) in Auckland, where I am currently Professor of Midwifery and Associate Dean of postgraduate research. We do not have children due to fertility issues and this has given me a certain perspective on childbirth and women's health issues and research. I resonate with Buddhist and Yogic understandings of leading a good and ethical life and align myself with approaches to inquiry that bring forth meaning – hence my passion for hermeneutic phenomenology. I started my research career using Grounded Theory, but when I met and spoke to Professor Liz Smythe over a cup of tea, I knew instantly I had come home to where I needed to be. I was fortunate to have Liz as my primary supervisor, who is now friend and mentor. I was also fortunate to have Dr Deb Spence as my second supervisor, who is an amazingly thoughtful Gadamerian hermeneut. Following my own PhD, examining the lived experiences of joy at childbirth, I conducted postdoctoral projects using phenomenology and now write and teach hermeneutic phenomenology with my co-editor Gill and supervise postgraduate research students using phenomenology. To do hermeneutic phenomenology is to penetrate beyond the natural attitude (see below); for me, this has been transformative and life enhancing.

I (Gill) am currently working as a Professor in Perinatal Health at the University of Central Lancashire (UCLan), located in North-West UK. I have three children, one to a former relationship and two to my current husband, with a more recent addition to our family of a granddaughter – Evie – what a joy. I started my undergraduate degree later in life (27 years) and am unusual in that all my degrees are from the university where I now work. This is in part due to the life circumstance of studying, working and being a single parent (and so limited travel was a bonus), and because all my studying at UCLan has been so wonderfully positive. My first two degrees are in psychology, and I then went onto complete a PhD in midwifery that focused on birth trauma; my first real introduction to qualitative research and philosophy. Moving from a quantitative, positivistic epistemology to a one that focuses on individual, subjective and emic perspectives was as challenging as it was rewarding. Hermeneutic phenomenology is without doubt a gift that keeps on giving – there is always more to learn, and most importantly brings me into contact with wonderful like-minded individuals whose goal is to uncover what it is to be human.

## Type of phenomenology

We are aware of the challenges of the neophyte phenomenologist when confronted with an array of different options. Many qualitative research methodologies focus on human experiences in different ways. Phenomenology is a genre of research focusing on lived experiences of the phenomenon. Other types of applied phenomenology include Interpretive Phenomenology Analysis (IPA), descriptive, lifeworld, phenomenological sociology, psychology and neurophenomenology to name a few. Our focus is on interpretive hermeneutic phenomenology. The greatest confusion seems to be in the distinction between IPA and hermeneutic phenomenology. We would concur with Zahavi (2019) when he states:

> Whereas the phenomenological orientations of Giorgi's [descriptive and more Husserlian] and van Manen's approaches are distinct and recognisable, the phenomenological origin and character of IPA is somewhat more questionable. The approach is clearly qualitative. It is non-reductive and seeks to provide rich experiential descriptions. But is it sufficient to simply consider the perspective of the agent/patient/client in order to make the approach in question phenomenological? .... Phenomenologically informed qualitative research has different aims than phenomenological philosophy, but it is questionable whether the former [IPA] can qualify as phenomenological if it either ignores or misinterprets the latter. (126)

This is not to infer IPA is "wrong" or "bad" but to simply say it is different from the hermeneutic phenomenology we have adopted. The phenomenological approach we use has an explicit ontological orientation underpinned by philosophical underpinnings that inform a method for health, social and educational research. However, we remain open to exploring these tensions and expanding our horizons of understanding. Sally Goldspink and Hilary Engward (2019) have written about what they term reflexive echoes in IPA and Virginia Eatough and Jonathan Smith (2008) have given a good overview of IPA describing it within a family of phenomenological psychology approaches. Both are valuable resources for those curious to read more about the differences and tensions between hermeneutic phenomenology and IPA approaches.

## Feeling the fear and jumping in anyway

The importance of not being constrained or bounded by predetermined rules can strike fear for some. Hermeneutic phenomenology is by its very ontological nature interpretive, always emergent and often hard to "pin down" to a set of fixed rules and processes. Any hermeneutic phenomenology project done well takes time and requires someone eager to engage in a thought-provoking challenging scholarly activity that is attuned to the dialectic.

The dialectic lies at the heart of hermeneutic phenomenology, inviting us to rethink our fascination with differences and conflicts – differences which often create false dichotomies and polemic beliefs. Instead, hermeneutic phenomeno-logical open us up to appreciating different worldviews and a willingness to be guided into a clearing where expanding horizons of understanding sheds light on our shared humanity. Gadamer describes the significance of horizons of understanding:

> The concept of 'horizon' suggests itself because it expresses the superior breadth of vision that the person who is trying to understand must have. To acquire a horizon means that one learns to look beyond what is close at hand – not in order to look away from it but to see it better.
>
> (Gadamer 1960/1975, 305)

Seeing the world "better" is about expanding and enriching our understanding when our present, contextual and historical horizon encounters new vistas of understanding – a process named a "fusion of horizons." Yet some horizons of understanding can be limiting, restrictive and closed. For example, you may encounter some "horizons of understanding" within yourself, in others or in groups, that close off possibilities – perhaps fixed understandings resulting from places of overt bias and fundamentalism and other forms of "isms" creating con-striction and limitation to further understanding. We have argued in a previous article that hermeneutic phenomenology is a political challenge to limiting and constrained modes of thinking and evidence (Thomson and Crowther 2019). Thus, to do this genre of research takes courage because it is often perceived as a deviant path away from the status quo of established empirical discourses (a particular horizon of understanding) beckoning us to yield to an ongoing process of new emergent understandings as we embrace a fusing of horizons. Likewise, working this way requires a unique attitude.

Adopting a hermeneutic phenomenological attitude attunes us to a wonder and questioning about what matters most; it speaks to the human yearning to understand the world we live and use tools and ideas (from our unique cos-mological, sociocultural and spiritual worldviews) to inform our approaches. The dialectic is thus more than a simple dialogue or conversation, to enter a dialectical process is to bring an awareness of possibilities in which a fusion of horizons (when we get "over our" "differences"). For example, in Aotearoa, New Zealand, Tangata whenua (literally the people of the land), collectively named "Māori" after colonisation, base their yearly Calendar on stars – in the Western world, this is based on the moon and sun cycles – yet, are we so different in our purposes? We love labelling everything and at times this can lead us to polemic thinking missing the existential whole meaning. This is where hermeneutic phenomenology offers an exciting way to do research – it brings an ontological focus that can never be complete, remains openly attuned to wonder and avoids reinforcing or forming further dichotomies that lends little to nothing to our understanding. We would contend that reaching through to what matters most in our shared humanness is so much more motivating.

Hermeneutic phenomenology helps us recover or refocus our work on individual or subjective lived experiences and leave behind the idea that objectifying human experience is possible or desirable. This work is about not splitting objectivity and subjectivity – it is about incorporating all that it means to be human in our contexts and life worlds. Husserl, the teacher and mentor of Heidegger, said that the natural and human sciences have tended to understand the world through the natural attitude rather than the experience as lived. A natural attitude is our pre-reflective orientation to the world where taken-for-granted everydayness remains the locality of our thinking and practice activity. Conversely, the phenomenological attitude is concerned with noticing what is previously taken-for-granted. A phenomenological attitude is not to be confused with bracketing out our preconceived ideas and beliefs (see below), but noticing them and seeing them in relation to whatever experience and phenomenon is calling on you to investigate. Put simply, to attune to a phenomenological attitude is about being attentive, thoughtful and open in our gaze whilst recognising that we already have our own fusion of horizon, which influences how we interpret the world.

Hermeneutic phenomenology is an attempt to ground us in our world through profound understanding of experience, consciousness and awareness. It provides an opportunity to be immersed in a methodological examination of lived experiences in a thoughtful, attentive and noticing manner to reveal what it means to be in the world. Being-in-the-world, according to Heidegger, is to orientate away from an objective mode challenging the idea of differences between inner and outer worlds. To continue to perceive an external world separate from ourselves maintains the idea of some transcendental split between the objective and subjective worlds. This view would maintain that it is possible to reduce the objective to "something" external to us so that "it" can be scrutinised and categorised in some way. For the hermeneutic researcher, this is an invitation to reflexively integrate from start to finish their open engagement with self, others and context – this requires courage, honesty and transparency.

Many times, in our courses, when participants share their journeys to hermeneutic phenomenology and present their projects, a certain mood permeates the group. As a participant shares their passion, the group palpably attunes to an emotive, provocative mood that at times triggers a confrontational realisation of self in response to the potency of the stories of human experience being shared. The shared resonance can be tangible, and for many of us, this may be the first occasion when such insights, feelings and thoughts about an aspect of human experience awaken in a conscious way. The honesty and trust that are built in such moments are deeply affecting and touch many of us profoundly. Avoiding this level of fully showing up and being touched is perhaps related to avoidance in seeing differently beyond the taken-for-granted status quo? For some of us, there may be a reluctance to fully show up as we continue to cover over what is being shared in normative language, idle talk and dominant discourses. Hermeneutic phenomenology calls us to remain open in our listening and any reluctance, conscious and unconscious, may result in a lost opportunity for advancing our human understanding.

This viewpoint or "natural attitude" would deny us the powerful moments of insights when a glimpse of our shared worlds is afforded by being fully there in our awareness of our interconnected totality. Husserl asserted that a positivistic reduction of science to mere facts leads to the loss or covering over of life's meanings. We have heard this sense of impasse due to the dominance of positivist reductionism expressed time and time again by health, education and social care researchers who seek to uncover meaning in their worlds of practice. Husserl cautions:

> The crisis of philosophy implies the crisis of all modern sciences as members of the philosophical universe: at first a latent theme, then more and more …
> (Husserl 1970/1936, 12)

If we want to change how we do things, we need to think differently, to adopt a phenomenological attitude, to attune in a way that is open and receptive; only then can we begin to understand how we do things and what meanings dwell within the experience. This is particularly important in health, social and educational research – a world in which the natural attitude is often privileged. Many that we listen to and meet through our work are deeply concerned with this growing sense of crisis of meaning in their fields, which eventually brings them to hermeneutic phenomenological projects. As you read the chapters, note each author's beckoning to this way of working in their pursuit of finding meaning. There is a perceptive mood of yearning that seeks to reach beyond the natural attitude and pose meaningful evocative questions through reflexive openness. Gadamer calls us to such opening in our questioning, "*The essence of the question is the opening up, and keeping open, of possibilities*" (1960/1975, 266). This speaks of an inclination to openness in our pursuit of research questioning in which hitherto covered over understandings reveal themselves through our own historicity[2] of understanding, "… *dialogue, [and] authentic exchange*" (Vandermause 2008, 70–71). Kent Smith, in chapter 12, provides valuable insights into this opening questioning and the way of attuning that honours the emergent and not yet emergent tension in the process of becoming a hermeneutic phenomenological researcher.

The philosophical underpinnings of hermeneutic phenomenological thinking are a persistent call to be reflexively attuned and open to new horizons of understanding. This way of scholarship safeguards the congruence of our interpretive leaps and leads to glimpses of depth and richness that gifts value to the reader. This is the ort[3] of this work, a locus or site where the foundational principle or essential dwelling place of the methodology is realised. It is the inspiration of this book.

## "Method" or "methodology"

Is hermeneutic phenomenology a method or methodology? This can confuse neophyte researchers in our experience and causes much confusion. The definitions in Figure 1.1 are adapted from Saks and Allsop (2019). Using these definitions, it

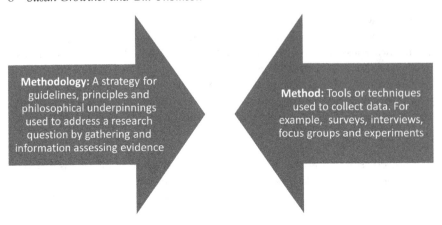

*Figure 1.1* Definitions of Methods and Methodology

is easy to see how hermeneutic phenomenology is a methodology rather than a method because it provides principles and guidelines through the application of philosophical underpinnings. It is an interpretive methodology that values and honours changing contexts, historicity and myriad perspectives. It is an ontological endeavour that acknowledges the embeddedness of our participants (including us as researchers) within worlds and their mutual and socially constructed understandings. Hermeneutic phenomenology draws upon a philosophical worldview and uses qualitative research design methods such as interviews (as well as other approaches such as body maps, see Helen and Elizabeth's Chapter 7).

## Hermeneutic phenomenology as applied methodology

The hermeneutic phenomenological methodology is used when the research question seeks meanings of a phenomenon that intends to disclose understanding of a human experience (Crist and Tanner 2003). Hermeneutics is the study of meanings, relationships and thinking upon relationships in context; it is not a study of objects separate from the whole (Gadamer 1960/1975). Hermeneutics seeks to explicate and reveal the inner meaning of human lived experiences and is the art, skill of interpreting and understanding of such meanings. Hermeneutics does not seek to classify or construct labels of phenomena but rather reveals the meanings of Being-there or Dasein as an ontological enquiry. Hermeneutics and phenomenology concern two modes or styles of questioning – the What and How:

- Phenomenological question: **What is the lived experience** *of reading a book?*
- Hermeneutic question: **How is the** *lived experience of reading a book* **meaningful?**

Inherent in questions of lived experience is a desire to reveal meaning (Dreyfus 1991). The purpose is not to generate theories, present generalisations or develop a way of predicting phenomena, rather, it is concerned with making sense of and understanding the different human ways of Being-in-the-world.

Hermeneutic phenomenology projects require an intimacy between the texts of the participants' lived experiences and the mind of the researcher or *"the bridging of personal or historical distance between minds"* (Gadamer 1976, 95). Gadamer adopted a more practical application of hermeneutic phenomenology. In his seminal works *Truth and Method* (1960/1975) and *Philosophical Hermeneutics* (2008/1967), Gadamer articulated a philosophical approach that highlighted the conditions through which understanding itself takes place. The "Phenomenology" and "Hermeneutics" of Heidegger and Gadamer underpin an evolving methodology that is invaluable when engaging in the quest of greater human understanding. Combined, they provide an opportunity to delve deeper into the human lived experience of life and illuminate meanings that may be forgotten through sustained exploration and questioning.

## A brief history of hermeneutic phenomenology

The phenomenological tradition is associated with several European philosophers stretching back to Hegel (1770–1831) and Brentano (1838–1917). However, it was Brentano's student Edmund Husserl (1859–1938) who is regarded as the father of phenomenology. Husserl contested the stance of the scientific community for not acknowledging the human experience. He claimed scientific endeavours of human behaviours produced artificial, superficial and de-contextualised findings. Husserl was the first philosopher to openly challenge the natural attitude of Cartesian mind-body dualism, and turned his focus on exploring how phenomena are revealed in consciousness (Husserl 2001). One of Husserl's pivotal ideas is that of intentionality in which consciousness is always being directed towards objects – whether real or perceived. Another Husserlian notion – bracketing or phenomenological reduction – concerns setting aside our preconceptions and pre-understandings of the focus of a study so that what can be described is the "true" essence of the phenomenon. Husserl's aim was to reach objectivity by removing outside variants and distractions of personal accounts. However, this belief was strongly contested by Heidegger, Husserl's student, as well as others.

Heidegger turned his focus from epistemological questions of knowing to ontology[4] and the study of being itself. He considered the only way in which we can understand the meaning and to understand phenomenon is via our lived experiences. He used the term *Dasein* (translated as Being-there), to describe how we as human beings are "open heads turned towards the world" whereby what we know and understand is inextricably related to our lifeworld (Sheenan 2000).

Unlike Husserl, Heidegger understood consciousness and the world as inseparable entities in an interconnected *Being-in-the-world*. Consciousness, for Heidegger, thus becomes interpreted as a historical constructed lived experience. For Heidegger, it is the situatedness of Being-in-the-world and the historicity of a person's background that allow for understanding the world from a certain point of view (Heidegger 1927/1962). It is therefore impossible for us to stand outside of what we know and to bracket our pre-understandings. The context for Heidegger is central to Being and is an inseparable part of the whole of our Being-in-the-world. Being and world are one and the same and represented in translation by the use of hyphens between words to signal this a priori interconnectedness.

To appreciate Being-in-the-world, it is necessary to understand Heidegger's interpretation of Dasein. Dasein is the kind of being (sometimes written with a capital "B" = Being) who understands that it exists and is shaped and informed by that understanding. It is a formal conception of existence, a human being – a being that I am myself, my mineness, my being – creating the possibility of authentic and inauthentic life. Likewise, Dasein is characterised by its historicity, meaning that Dasein is constituted by its past experience in the world, whether a Dasein is conscious of this or not. Being-in-the-world is, therefore, the grounding or foundational state of Being – a state in which Dasein stands. It is a unifying phenomenon that signals that Dasein and world are not separate but are always already together with no internal and external divide. Significantly, Being-in-the-world as Dasein reveals concern towards the world –and is only possible because of Dasein's Being-in-the-world. Moreover, the concern is undifferentiated ontologically – Heidegger did not assign a value laden on the term concern, but rather his position is that what we are concerned with in the world is fundamentally based on who we are.

Therefore, to bracket or in some way to attempt, as a researcher, to separate our understandings from their contexts and our own pre-understandings is unachievable. As Koch (1996) explains, there is an indissoluble unity between the world and people. Our lives professionally and personally are always already with us in the world. Likewise, chapter authors and you as a reader are similarly always already in an indissoluble unity with the world. The traditions of phenomenology and hermeneutics are themselves in and of the world. Furthermore, they are not stationary; they come from a rich and textual thinking history that continues to evolve. Gadamer (1960/1975), Heidegger's student, maintained that such methodology is not fixed but continually open to new insights and possibilities.

## Phenomenology

Phenomenology is an invitation to observe and collect data pertaining to people's experience of life world phenomena. It is a method for uncovering what lies hidden. Phenomenology is descriptive, focussing on the structures of experience and seeks to surface meanings of lived experiences (van Manen 1997). In the process, feeling-based understandings are brought into text form, helping the invisible become visible (Kvale and Brinkman 2009). Heideggerian phenomenology is fundamentally about Being and not about theories, ideas and problem-solving. Phenomenology is, at its core, an investigation and focus on experiences as lived in and lived through.

## Lived experience

The core of hermeneutic phenomenology as a research method is the lived experience of something. These experiences are first person contextually and temporally situated, pre-reflexive taken for granted activities and encounters in everyday life. They are lived through in a natural attitude harbouring unrevealed meanings. The focus is on experience as lived rather than something already perceived, considered, interpreted, characterised and represented. People's lived experiences in health, social and educational practice are invaluable because they can inform sustainable and acceptable care planning, treatment interventions, educational approaches leading to improvements in care, safety and satisfaction with services.

## Phenomenon

The phenomenon, according to Heidegger, is that which is essentially withdrawn, hidden, forgotten, covered up and even disguised (Heidegger 1927/1962). Phenomena are always covered over and can never be completely uncovered. They are taken-for-granted in pre-reflective and unnoticed within lived experiences. To examine and bring to awareness the unnoticed in lived experiences fully is never possible and is always an on the way, an un-concealing.

Phenomena can reveal themselves as **appearance** which is as close to the thing in itself as we ever get, such as crying with sadness when a friend dies. This is a hint of background sadness, yet the phenomenon of sadness itself is not entirely revealed. The sadness can also **announce** itself such as through observing the tears, or the phenomenon can show itself as **semblance** when what seems to be sadness may, in fact, be representing something else. For example, the tears could be from fatigue and relief because the friend had a long protracted difficult illness. Although a phenomenon is never fully revealed, it can be unconcealed by adopting a phenomenological attitude and illuminating that which eludes. For the hermeneutic phenomenologist, the task is to thematise a phenomenon of interest and bring it into language. In this way, our studies foreground phenomenon from lived-experience descriptions illuminating phenomena that were hidden and just out of reach into words (prose and/or poetry) and other art forms. For example, see Polly's use of poetry to give voices to children in Chapter 3. To thematise the phenomenon is the endeavour which seeks ways to bring to light phenomena which are hidden within lived experiences so that they can show themselves, as themselves, from themselves. To go to the lived experience is the opportunity to uncover what is concealed and expand our horizons of understanding.

## Philosophical underpinnings that inform Hermeneutic phenomenology

At the heart of quality hermeneutic phenomenology is reflexivity and the application of philosophical notions that not only underpin methodological decisions but also help foreground, surface and reveal phenomena. One participant who attended our course asked: "so how many philosophical notions do you need to do this work?" Great question, which got us thinking. We would contend that there are fundamental notions needed to form the foundation of a robust hermeneutic phenomenology study so that we can orientate and attune to an ontological project that moves beyond description and ontical concerns.[5] Notions such as Dasein and Being-there and Being-in-the-world, for example, are key underpinning ontological considerations to our work – these help frame research designs based on knowledge of how our research participants (and self) are historical, contextual, situated human beings that have their own unique horizon of understanding. This is what we need to consider as we engage in reflexive practices and what we aim to tap into when we explore their lived accounts.

Other philosophical and, indeed, wider theoretical notions, as you will read in the following chapters, will come into play as the data (the gathering of understanding) and horizons of understandings fuse into a new way of seeing as the phenomenon shows itself. We consider the following list as tentative foundational notions "to set the scene," **not** a definitive list but simply a guide to reading/ learning as a "way in" to health, social and educational research. Some have already been discussed in this chapter.

- Ontic and ontological
- Aletheia (see below)
- Dasein
- Being-in-the-world
- Horizons of understanding and fusion of horizons
- Forestructures of understanding[6]
- Hermeneutic circle/spiral[7]

Most of the above list are used in many of the chapters to follow; other notions in the following chapters include:

- Attunement – Chapters 2 and 12
- Thrownness – Chapters 3 and 6
- Technology, parts and pieces – Chapter 4
- Being-towards-death – Chapter 4
- the They and idle talk – Chapter 5
- Authenticity – Chapters 5 and 11
- Ready-to-hand and unready-to-hand – Chapters 4, 6 and 12
- Embodiment/lived body – Chapter 7
- Fourfold – Chapter 8
- Care – Chapter 9
- Having-been-ness – Chapter 10
- In-seeing – Chapter 12
- Clearing – Chapter 12

Authors refer to multiple notions in their chapters – this list signals some of the main notions they refer to.

How to know which notions to use and which philosophers (or other theorists) to help make the interpretive leap? This is not easy to answer. The two pieces of advice we would proffer are as follows:

- first align with hermeneutic phenomenology as an ontological project by reading seminal writers in this area to understand its philosophical underpinning orientation, to awaken a mood or wonder and acknowledge that this orientation and attunement brings into focus an epistemological, ontological and axiological understanding. This is building your theoretical framework and will guide you.

- second, let the data (gathered understandings) guide you in your reading, for example, if you hear stories of shame, joy, redemption, then read other work that has this as its focus – find the philosophers and theorists that best resonate with your work/projects and illuminate the phenomenon of interest.

Whilst this can be a lot of reading and pondering, and it may take you down blind alleys and rabbit holes, this is about learning how to think thinking, a process that opens possibilities yet unknown. As you engage and embrace these two pieces of advice, your projects will draw you further than your natural attitude and the taken-for-granted into a deeper phenomenological attitude where meanings will reveal themselves in unexpected ways. This can be unfamiliar territory to some newbie hermeneutics phenomenologists who find themselves concerned about finding the "right" meaning and concluding a study with a final "truth" about how it is.

## Meaning and truth

Meaning is everywhere, in all our experiences, and these experiences always have multiple layers of significance which are constantly emerging. This points to a relational totality of meaningfulness that permeates human life, including that of ourselves as researchers. It is this "meaning" that hermeneutic phenomenology attunes to and poses the question "where does this meaning come from?" and if we seek to report such meaning in our research, "what is the final correct meaning?" But caution is required here because this draws us into a further discussion about the notion of adequacy. The idea that a final correct meaning exists, or establishing an absolute truth is an anathema to the philosophy of hermeneutic phenomenology.

In hermeneutic phenomenology, we are not seeking an absolute concrete truth, a provable testimony but instead an unconcealedness, a disclosure or a revealing of a phenomenon on the way to further understanding. Unconcealing (Aletheia) gestures the idea that there has been a forgetfulness, a hiddenness and concealment. This is different to veritas – a form of truth or testimony that may be a verifiable fixed essential truth. An aletheia orientation to truth releases us from the burden of establishing the final answer to our questions and invites an unconcealing on the way to knowing. Instead, we recognise that truth is always in a play of concealing and unconcealing as new interpretations emerge. In previous articles, we have explored the hypocrisy and futility of attempting to claim a final or complete meaning applying insights from Gadamer, Derrida and Ricouer (see Crowther and Thomson 2020, Crowther et al. 2017).

In the following chapters, authors show you how existential phenomenological notions provide inroads into revealing the meanings within and around everyday experiences of their interest areas illuminating the "how" of practices – often in unexpected, creative and surprising ways. However, this can be risky because the path is not marked clearly on any map – moreover, it is often advisable to get off the track most used and discover new clearings! Feeling the fear of the unboundedness of a methodology that has no fixed lineal strategies can be daunting – but jumping in any way can be exhilarating, surprising and transformative.

## Interpretive leaps

The analysis of data collected is through description and interpretation whilst remaining reflexively attuned and remaining open to interpretive leaps. We published an article to present "a way" of moving towards interpretive work and the interpretive leap (Crowther and Thomson 2020). The following two figures come from that article. In Figure 1.2, a simplified diagrammatic representation of three levels is suggested to illustrate the need in hermeneutic phenomenology to move beyond description alone.

We acknowledge that this is always a work in progress and cannot be taken as the final complete "methods foundation" for all hermeneutic phenomenology studies. Although presented in a lineal way, the experience is often a lot "messier" and more iterative. However, it provides a beginning template for discussion and gestures to the ort of this work. Figure 1.3 builds on Figure 1.2, providing a further visual representation of an iterative journey – parts to whole, whole to parts and so forth.

The following chapters bring to life through myriad examples of what these diagrams gesture to. For most of us bringing ideas into examples is hugely beneficial. We all find our own unique individual way as our projects evolve and gather understandings, vis-vis., it is the data which reveals novel ways to proceed. As Husserl and Heidegger remind us, we need to constantly return to the thing itself so that the thing (phenomenon) itself can show itself from itself. This cannot be rushed. Kent, in Chapter 12, reminds us that the experience of doing hermeneutic phenomenological research is one of courage and a special journey to savour and love.

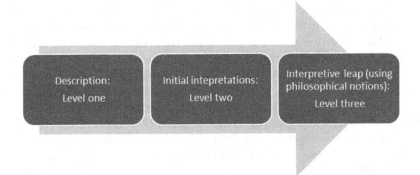

*Figure 1.2* Three Levels

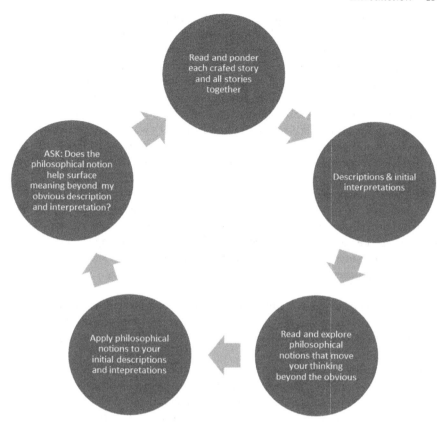

*Figure 1.3* Circular Repetition of the Interpretive Process

## How to read Heidegger

As you begin to read Hermeneutic phenomenological literature, especially the seminal works of Heidegger and others, we want to share some advice. We are not intending to matriculate you into a course on philosophy in this book. Our mission here is guiding you towards ways of knowing and thinking so that you can apply hermeneutic phenomenology in your projects. We appreciate that reading Heideggerian texts for the first time can be a frustrating and an overwhelming experience. George Steiner (1991) describes the experience of reading Heidegger's texts: *"We are to be slowed down, bewildered, and barred in our reading so that we may be driven deep"* (8). Heidegger's writings call us into a space, into a clearing where we can ponder deeply and dwell in wonder as "long-buried" meanings surface and become illuminated. However, the language and complex word usage can trip us up.

For Heidegger, language is often an instrument – a bit like the finger that points to the moon, it is not the moon itself but a gesturing towards. In his writings, there is a lot of etymologising of German and Greek words (that is, going back to the original historical meanings of words). Susan keeps an etymology dictionary and thesaurus nearby when writing. The significance of language, tradition and history in Heidegger's writings cannot be underestimated. At times Heidegger takes a passage, for example, from Heraclitus, Kant or Nietzsche and excavates from them individual syllables, words, or phrases and interprets their original, long-buried or eroded wealth of meaning. He then demonstrates that the occlusion of this meaning has in some way been altered and perhaps even damaged by subsequent Western thought. Heidegger's work reminds us that language and words can be revisited, rediscovered and restored – in doing so we can bring an intellectual renascence and renewed moral possibility to our interpretive work.

Without a doubt many of us get frustrated by texts which seem so incomprehensible. First, do not be in a hurry to read through Heidegger at the same speed you read other texts. Second, do not read once and expect to "fully" appreciate the message being conveyed. As Steiner (1991) suggests, perhaps Heidegger did not want to be merely "understood" in the customary sense. Heidegger wants to take us on a journey of thinking,

> Do not be in too great a hurry to get to the end of Heraclitus the Ephesian's book; the path is hard to travel. Gloom is there and darkness devoid of light. But if an initiate be your guide, the path shines brighter than sunlight. (11)

Initiation in this context is not concerned with understanding in the ordinary sense – this is about accepting entry into an alternative order or space of meaning and of being – of attuning to an attitude of wonder and openness. The invitation is to gaze beyond what we conceive of things and take a leap of faith out of our current ways of knowing.

For us reading Heidegger is an "experiencing" of something strange and uncanny that, when we are ready, draws us into acceptance. We would urge you to suspend your conventions of common logic and unexamined grammar in order to commune with the texts so that they may shine light into new ways of knowing. This involves embracing the challenge of reading something that, on the first read, seems totally unintelligible – believe us – we have been there! Sometimes the language reads in a clumsy way, an overly verbose way and exasperating erudite way; sometimes, the grammar and syntax simply do not work, and the flow jars us. At times you can find yourself grasping at elusive insights that are just out of reach as you read – keep going, you are often on the threshold of something – take notes, record your thoughts.

With time, comprehension grows as you read secondary sources and seminal works. To read Heidegger is to enter a dialectic with the author – to read and re-read texts brings understanding and ontological insights that inform your studies. This is a whole new way of reading, thinking and engaging with research – be patient with yourself. You are in the process of opening new vistas of understanding, and you may have to stumble over challenging terrains to get the view. Let go of cause-and-effect relationships – let go of a priori notions, concepts and repackaged theoretical professional frameworks. Return to what matters most as you read Heidegger and remain open to the play within his texts. He does not gift us a way out of our contemporary concerns; his own life story is a testament to that. If you read about his life, you will see his own political activities were appalling choices.[8] What his writings gift are a plethora of thinking that has evoked a whole tradition of thinking differently. The invitation is to read with openness, not about "getting it" in any concrete way. To read Heidegger is to embark on a journey one small step at a time. More suggestions:

- When you read a passage of text, always return to it later and re-read it making a note of confusing passages or of those which seem particularly relevant to your work.
- Read secondary literature on Heidegger's philosophy – they often provide useful commentary on how a particular idea in Heidegger's work speaks to the work of other philosophers.
- Remember, the original Heideggerian texts were written in German – consider translation issues – seek out other translations that may help you better understand a philosophical notion.
- Ontological descriptions are challenging in language and often require new words and new conflated or re-constructed words, as well as the use of hyphens, capitals and non-capitals.
- Read the work of others who have applied ontological notions in their studies – the chapters in this book will help.
- Join or start a local Heideggerian reading group – we have both done this in our own institutions. Through a group, reading understanding comes and surprising insights arise.

Liz Smythe and Deb Spence wrote a wonderful article about reading Heidegger, which provides further instruction on how to navigate these texts. They used the experiences of their own postgraduate students to show the variety of ways of engaging with Heidegger's writing. They discuss the importance of attuning in the right way that something will stick as you persevere and the gift of the struggle bringing insights hoped for, they conclude:

> To read Heidegger is to open oneself to an experience that may well become life transforming. To learn to do that means becoming patient, careful, attentive and humble. No one else can teach you how to "be" in such a mood; it must be granted the time and opportunity to "come."
>
> (Smythe and Spence 2020, 8)

To read more of Liz and Deb's, refer to Chapter 2. Through the chapters, you will read how each author came to an appreciation of the philosophical texts and found ways to apply them to their studies and take interpretive leaps in their analysis. Each one traversed their own struggles and persevered until insights surfaced that illuminated the phenomena of their concerns.

## How to read this book

The authors make up an international cohort of hermeneutic phenomenology researchers who explore a multitude of phenomena in health and social care and education. Each author(s) proffers a unique perspective, a variety of methodological choices and uses different philosophical notions to underpin, illuminate and interpret their findings. Reflexivity is crucial in this genre of research and is central to all chapters. Some authors have a more philosophical leaning than others and take us on a journey of unravelling the philosophical underpinnings in the context of their research journey – others take a more prosaic approach to the philosophy.

All authors were provided with the same guidance template for their chapters, yet what emerged was so much more than the "bounded" constraints of our original "please include" list. As co-editors, we have endeavoured to ensure congruence and flow through the chapters whilst delighting and honouring how they attune to their writing and bring forth their own distinct presentation. As a guide, each chapter begins by situating the topic and presenting background information of how the philosophical underpinnings and orientation have been taken up in their research in relation to hermeneutic phenomenology. Moreover, the focus of each chapter is on praxis, moving from theory and conceptions to doing the research itself. What you will discover is that each author has their own journey into hermeneutic phenomenological scholarship. Each reveals how they found the journey worthwhile yet requiring trust in the process and determination. Likewise, how hermeneutic phenomenology researchers address the rigour in their projects is important. In our final chapter, we reflect on the chapters and reflect on how we can attune to trustworthiness in hermeneutic phenomenology research scholarship.

You may decide to read cover to cover in a lineal fashion – you may dip in and out through the chapters as they pull your attention. You may go back and forth as your horizons of understanding expand and fuse with those of the authors. Each chapter holds insightful gems which we know you will enjoy. Enjoy the dialectic play between you and the authors as you journey through this reading and pondering. Reading hermeneutic phenomenology is an invitation to think differently and savour what is being glimpsed. Our final word of advice – gift yourself the time, this is about slow reading, noticing and creating moments to contemplate as you dialogue with the words and turn the pages.

## Notes

1. Praxis – praxis in this context is the practical application of doing hermeneutic phenomenology. In contrast, practice is the repetition of an activity to develop or/ and improve skills.
2. Historicity – Gadamer contends that no understanding is independent of socio-cultural factors vis-à-vis., any ideas, thoughts and beliefs are conditioned and informed by historical contexts and situations. In other words, our understandings are developed and influenced over time as such any claim to truth is understood in a particular historical context.

3. To read and learn more about the term "Ort" beyond the everyday German meaning, see Heidegger, M. 1996. *The principle of reason*. Indiana: Indiana University Press.
4. Ontology – Concerned with being, the study of being. This lies at the heart of any hermeneutic phenomenology project.
5. Ontical/Ontic – Entities present-at-hand within the world in ways that can be categorised, measured and defined. Entities that are understood by Dasein as not being Dasein yet matter to Dasein. Can be the facts of something and the labels applied to things.
6. The fore-structure of understanding is constituted of a threefold structure: fore-having, fore-sight, and fore-conception. These are involved in all our interpretations and understanding and are a foundational part of Heidegger's ontological appreciation of how we come to know anything. You will see examples of these in the following chapters.
7. Hermeneutic circle/spiral – the dynamic and iterative process of understanding (usually text). The circle infers the idea that our understanding as a whole is established by reference to the individual parts, our own understanding and the whole in a to and fro dialectic. In other words, the whole text understanding and individual parts are always already understood through and by reference to one another. In this process, all interpretation and understanding are within cultural, historical, social and literary contexts and relates to our historicity (see endnote 2 above). Spiral is often used to indicate that we never arrive back to where we began, which may be symbolised by a closed circle.
8. A good source to examine some of Heidegger's political and anti-Semitic choices, see Mitchell, Andrew J., and Peter Trawny, eds. 2017. *Heidegger's black notebooks: Responses to anti-Semitism*. Columbia: Columbia University Press.

## References

Crist, J.D., and C.A. Tanner. 2003. "Interpretation/analysis methods in hermeneutic interpretive phenomenology." *Nursing Research* 52 (3):202–205.

Crowther, S., P. Ironside, D. Spence, and L. Smythe. 2017. "Crafting stories in hermeneutic phenomenology research: A methodological device." *Qualitative Health Research* 27 (6):826–835. doi: 10.1177/1049732316656161.

Crowther, S., and G. Thomson. 2020. "From description to interpretive leap: Using philosophical notions to unpack and surface meaning in hermeneutic phenomenology research." *International Journal of Qualitative Methods* 19. doi: 10.1177/1609406920969264.

Dibley, L., S. Dickerson, M. Duffy, and R. Vandermause. 2020. *Doing hermeneutic phenomenological research: A practical guide*: Thousand Oaks, CA: SAGE Publications Limited.

Dreyfus, H.L. 1991. *Being-in-the-world: A commentary on Heidegger's Being and time, division I*. Cambridge, MA: MIT Press.

Eatough, V., and J.A. Smith. 2008. "Interpretative phenomenological analysis." *The Sage Handbook of Qualitative Research in Psychology* 179:194.

Gadamer, H.G. 1960/1975. *Truth and method*. Translated and edited by G. Barden and J. Cumming. New York: Seabury.

Gadamer, H.G. 1976. *Philosophical hermeneutics*. Berkeley: University of California Press.

Gadamer, H.G. 2008/1967. *Philosophical hermeneutics*. Translated and edited by D.E. Linge. London: University of California Press.

Goldspink, S., and H. Engward. 2019. "Booming clangs and whispering ghosts: Attending to the reflexive echoes in IPA research." *Qualitative Research in Psychology* 16 (2):291–304. doi: 10.1080/14780887.2018.1543111.

Heidegger, M. 1927/1962. *Being and time*. Translated by J. Macquarrie and E. Robinson. New York: Harper.

Heidegger, M., 1996. *The principle of reason*. Indiana: Indiana University Press.

Heidegger, M. 1995. *Being and time*. Oxford: Basil Blackwell.

Husserl, E. 1970/1936. *The crisis of European sciences and transcendental phenomenology*. Evanston: North Western University Press.

Husserl, E. 2001. *Logical investigations*. Translated by D. Moran. London: Routledge.

Koch, T. 1996. "Implementation of a hermeneutic inquiry in nursing: Philosophy, rigour and representation." *Journal of Advanced Nursing* 24:174–184.

Kvale, S., and S. Brinkman. 2009. *InterViews: Learning the craft of qualitative research interviewing*. London: Sage Publications.

Mitchell, A.J. and P. Trawny. eds., 2017. *Heidegger's black notebooks: Responses to antisemitism*. Columbia: Columbia University Press.

Paley, J. 2016. *Phenomenology as qualitative research: A critical analysis of meaning attribution*. London: Routledge.

Saks, M., and J. Allsop. 2019. "Introduction to researching health." In *Researching health: qualitative, quantitative and mixed methods*, edited by M. Saks and J. Allsop. 1–3. London: Sage.

Sheenan, T. 2000. "Kehre and Ereignis: A prolegomenon to introduction to metaphysics." In *A companion to Martin Heidegger's introduction to metaphysics*, edited by G. Fried and R. Polt, 3–16. New Haven: Yale University Press.

Smythe, E. 2011. "From beginning to end: how to do hermeneutic interpretive phenomenology." In *Qualitative research in midwifery and childbirth: Phenomenological approaches*, edited by G. Thomson, F. Dykes and S. Downe, 35–54. London: Routledge.

Smythe, E. and D. Spence. 2020. Reading Heidegger. *Nursing Philosophy*, 21(2): e12271.

Steiner, G. 1991. *Martin Heidegger*. Chicago: University of Chicago Press.

Thomson, G., and S. Crowther. 2019. "Phenomenology as a political position within maternity care." *Nursing Philosophy* e12275.

Thomson, G., F. Dykes, and S. Downe, eds. 2011. *Qualitative research in midwifery and childbirth: Phenomenological approaches*. London: Routledge.

van Manen, M. 1997. "From meaning to method." *Qualitative Health Research* 7 (3):345–369. doi: 10.1177/104973239700700303.

van Manen, M. 2014. *Phenomenology of practice: Meaning-giving methods in phenomenological research and writing*. Walnut Creek, CA: Left Coast Press.

Vandermause, R.K. 2008. "The poiesis of the question in philosophical hermeneutics: Questioning assessment practices for alcohol use disorders." *International Journal of Qualitative Studies on Health and Well-being* 3 (2):68–76. doi: 10.1080/17482620801939584.

Wilcke, M. 2002. "Hermeneutic phenomenology as a research method in social work." *Currents: Scholarship in the Human Services* 1 (1):1–10.

Zahavi, D. 2019. "Applied phenomenology: why it is safe to ignore the epoché." *Continental Philosophy Review* 1–15.

# 2 Nurturing a spirit of attuning-to

*Liz Smythe and Deb Spence*

## Abstract

Heideggerian hermeneutic phenomenological methodology requires a spirit of attunement. Heidegger calls it "the way." It is a way of being, a listening, a wondering, that once grasped, stays with one through life's ongoing journey. This chapter draws on data from a study conducted with doctoral students engaged in hermeneutic phenomenological research. Through drawing on their experience, we seek to show how "the way" develops. We talk of the pre-understandings interview, recognising that the reflexivity evoked in such a conversation needs to continue through to the very end of the research, and beyond. Interviews with participants can be guided by a pre-thought set of questions, but it is attunement to being-there that matters.

## Introduction

Heideggerian hermeneutic phenomenological methodology requires a spirit of attunement. Heidegger calls it "the way." It is a way of being, a listening, a wondering, that once grasped, stays with one through life's ongoing journey. This chapter draws on data from a study conducted with doctoral students engaged in hermeneutic phenomenological research. Through drawing on their experience, we seek to show how "the way" develops. We talk of the pre-understandings interview, recognising that the reflexivity evoked in such a conversation needs to continue through to the very end of the research, and beyond. Interviews with participants can be guided by a pre-thought set of questions, but it is attunement to being-there that matters. Working with the transcripts is so much more than seeking to identify themes. It is a listening, a wondering, a releasement to the thoughts that come. Writing the thesis is not to write a report. It is rather to lose oneself in the thinking to the extent that the writing almost seems to write itself. Throughout this entire process, there is attunement to the writings of Heidegger, Gadamer, and other related philosophers. This chapter seeks to point to the way of attuning-to, always questioning, always wondering. Such a way of being underpins the spirit of staying methodologically congruent.

DOI: 10.4324/9781003081661-2

> You must note
> the way the soap dish enables you,
> or the window latch grants you freedom.
> Alertness is the hidden discipline of familiarity.
> From: Everything is waiting for you
> (Whyte, 2007, 361)

To come to a hermeneutic phenomenological study is to come with a sense that "everything is waiting for you." In the midst of a pandemic, the soap dish draws concerned attention when it is missing. The window latch meanwhile goes by unnoticed as the window is thrown open to call to a friend. To come to appreciate the everydayness of being, to notice those moments and things which are taken for granted yet "matter," requires what the poet David Whyte calls "alertness." Yet, what draws one to notice? What happens in the instant when one sees "as if for the first time"? In that seeing, how does understanding "come"? And as one exclaims "ahh," how then is such insight captured in language that enables others to share the gift of "seeing"? When, as a hermeneutic phenomenological researcher, one sits at one's desk dwelling with a transcript that describes an experience, how does the drawing-in of alertness propel one's thinking? How does one engage in wonder? In this chapter, drawing on the experiences of doctoral students, we track how they talked about attuning-to from their pre-understandings interview through to writing up their findings. We call it "the way" of researching in this methodological approach.

## Attuning-to

We have chosen to use the term 'attuning-to' as the pointer to describe that which we seek to reveal. It is to be alert, to heed one's mood, to tune-in to that which speaks, to let one's thoughts be free to wonder, to strive to bring such felt-knowing into language. It is a way of being/doing hermeneutic/phenomenological research that is so much more than any one term can convey (Smythe & Spence, 2020). van Manen (2014) describes how attuning provokes wonder:

> Wonder is that moment of being when one is overcome by awe or perplexity – such as when something familiar has turned profoundly unfamiliar, when our gaze has been drawn by the gaze of something that stares back at us. (360)

Heidegger wrestled with the challenge of languaging our experience of being (Heidegger, 1962). Those who translated his German to English struggled again. In the Macquarrie and Robinson (M&R) translation of *Being and Time* (1962), the page that first mentions "attunement" contains lengthy footnotes. They make the relevant translation as: "*What we indicate ontologically by the term 'state of mind' is ontically the most familiar and everyday sort of thing; our mood, our Being-attuned*" (172). They translate the German word *Befindlichkeit* as "state-of-mind" telling us there is no English word equivalent. Kisiel (2002, 67) draws attention to Stambaugh's translation of *Being and Time* in which she translates

*Befindlichkeit* as "attunement." "'Attunement' is far superior to the psychologically tinged 'state of mind' by far the worst blunder made in M&R (translation)." Kisiel explains: "*Befindlichkeit fully translated refers to how one 'finds oneself disposed, situated, positioned in and by the world*'" (68). For the hermeneutic phenomenological researcher this is a very different perspective from assuming a position of a neutral, objective researcher removed from any influence on or by the data collection process. We assert, "attuning-to" means one must be "in" the world of the research, not by careful planning but by finding oneself in a moment of happening. As such, in an interview, for example, one both influences the story being told and is influenced by the telling. It is an experience of immersion, of letting go, of soaking-up and awaiting the insights that come.

Back to M&R *Being and Time* footnotes; "Being-attuned" is expanded as *die Stimming, das Gestimmtsein.*" The noun "*'Stimmung' originally means the tuning of a musical instrument ... We shall usually translate it as 'mood'...'as having a mood*'" (172). Gelvin (1970, 78) furthers this discussion: "*One lives in or out of 'tune' with the world; and the variations of such tuning are moods.*" Heidegger (1962) makes it clear that we are never without moods. Our attuning awakens us to our mood of interest, or boredom, or frustration, drawing us in or turning us away. Moods reveal "how we find ourselves" in this interview, in this reading, in this attempt to write. "Attuning-to" picks up our mood and, in doing so, draws us back from the ontological experience of immersion to ontically examine and name: "*I am feeling excited by what I am hearing/reading/writing.*" Heidegger's (1962, 176) writing is translated into English as: "*Dasein's openness to the world is constituted existentially by the attunement of a state-of-mind.*" We could re-language that as "Being-as-researcher means being open to whatever situation I find myself in, and always attuning to 'how I find my mood'."

Heidegger (1962) further tells us that our being is influenced by what "*can matter to it*" (176). The researcher listens to the stories being told by the participant, attuned to what they perceive to matter in relation to the research question. Thus, some stories excite, while other stories feel irrelevant. Mood shapes the researcher's response in a manner that is felt rather than determined. What *matters* is what "calls" one's interest, which comes both from within (one's own agenda) and from without (the power of the story itself). Heidegger wrote:

> The call is not something which is explicitly performed by me, but that rather 'it' does the calling ... It calls, even though it gives the concernfully curious ear nothing to hear which might be passed along in further retelling and talked about in public.
>
> (Heidegger, 1962, 320–322)

Therefore, what matters, what captures one's attention (or not) comes first as mood. The hermeneutic phenomenological researcher needs then to discern the meaning behind the mood. What called? What matters? What might that mean? Or, taking on the notion of *Befindlichkeit* (Heidegger, 1962, 172), how do I find myself feeling/faring[1] amidst this experience?

Returning to the notion of *Stimmung*, Gadamer offers a discussion on music:

> … in the case of music, whether one makes music oneself, 'follows the notes' as we say, or if one only listens along with the music as it is played, it is all there – the repetition, variation, inversion, resolution – and it is precisely prescribed in advance. But only if one goes along with it, be it as a musical performer or be it as listener, does it come forward and one receives it. Otherwise it sweeps by and seems empty.
>
> (Gadamer, 2006a, 75)

Such is the nature of attuning-to. One is caught up, immersed in something much more than a series of notes. Further, Gadamer explains that interpretation is not just playing the correct musical notes, nor is reading about mere reproduction of words. "*Whoever truly makes music does not just spell it out by the notes: an interpreter in truth is the fulfiller of the music in such a way that it comes forth*" (Gadamer, 2006a, 77). That is the challenge of hermeneutic phenomenological research, to bring the meaning "forth." Gadamer warns us: "*reaching an understanding is a process that must succeed or fail in the medium of language*" (Gadamer, 2006b, 13). And that: "*Language deserts us, and it deserts us precisely because what enlightens is standing so strongly before our ever more encompassing gaze that words would not be adequate to grasp it*" (14).

Such is the challenge of hermeneutic phenomenology. It requires a way of being, an alertness, and attuning-to. It requires an appreciation that the way is shaped by mood, that one must immerse in the flow of unfolding. It is to glimpse. Such tentative, fleeting "seeing" brings the challenge of revealing when one is only vaguely sure of what one is trying to say and struggles to find the words that will share that which was glimpsed. In this chapter, we present "words" from doctoral students immersed in a hermeneutic phenomenological journey as they sought to language the nature of their experience. In this chapter, we ask the more specific question "what is the experience of attuning-to within hermeneutic phenomenological research?" In doing so, we ponder how attuning to our mood, how we are faring, shapes our understanding and subsequent interpretations as we make our way through our research projects.

## The way of the research

We did our own hermeneutic phenomenological doctoral research in the 1990s inspired by Professor Nancy and John Diekelmann. They led us to reading the philosophical writings of Heidegger and Gadamer. We came to grasp that one had to learn to trust the emerging way of going-forth. Over subsequent years we have supervised many doctoral students on similar pathways. As we move into retirement, we sensed our responsibility to capture the insights we had learnt through ours and others journeying. Our initial research question was "what is the experience of doing hermeneutic phenomenological research?" We gained ethics approval with agreement that past and current doctoral students could participate. In terms of current students, we argued that as supervisors, we were not examining their work; it went to external examiners. Further, we knew that these students were keen to have the opportunity to reflect on how their "way" had emerged. Fourteen interviews were conducted. It was mutually agreed to honour the participants (all of whom have now graduated) by naming them and including a link to their theses. Two publications have arisen (Smythe & Spence 2019; 2020) which shed light on the struggle and gift of reading philosophy, and the way of working with the data. Writing the two publications took us closer to that which we now name as "attuning to." The opportunity to write this book chapter enabled us to ponder afresh, to look with alert eyes for the nature of attuning. We started by laying out the crafted stories[2] in the chronological order from the beginning of the research process to the writing up of the thesis. We then examined them more thoughtfully, pondering how they revealed "attuning to." This is a different process from being guided by the data itself. Drawing on insights gained in earlier writing, we adopted a specific lens to illuminate how "attuning to" was revealed in the data. Any story about doing ontological hermeneutic phenomenological research is likely to reveal "attuning-to." Attuning, as we will discuss later, is one of Heidegger's existentialia[3] (Heidegger, 1962).

The methodology in this chapter is more hermeneutic than phenomenological. Participants tended to reflect on their experiences rather than tell a specific story. There are glimpses of being caught up in the ontological moment, interpreted through a more ontic lens of seeking to language "what happened." In writing this chapter, we seek to interpret the data in a manner that "shows" and lets learning come (Heidegger, 1968). We are mindful that we shared the journey with these doctoral students, thus our proud "knowing" of them colours our interpretations. Seeking to maintain a trustworthiness, drafts of this writing have gone back to the participants whose data we have drawn from, to gain their phenomenological nod, the unspoken nod of resonance that comes when the listener unthinkingly nods their affirmation (van Manen, 1990). We now turn to the accounts of doctoral students who found their own way along the hermeneutic phenomenological journey.

## GLIMPSING ATTUNING-TO

### Attuning to hermeneutic phenomenology

Our experience has taught us that some people are more suited to hermeneutic phenomenology than others. Getting that fit right at the start is key to the ongoing experience. Kent looks back on his choice:

> Choosing phenomenology as methodology doesn't feel traditional. It feels as though there's ability to be poetic, evocative, utilise language in different ways. And so that felt like a permission giving space.

Something drew Kent to a phenomenological approach. He came to it relishing the freedom to break free of tight strictures and explore ideas, writing styles and to let the experience itself be his guide. In each of the three sentences above he uses the word "feel/felt." Perhaps by the time of the interview, he was more aware of the feeling nature of his journey, yet in looking back, it seems he acknowledges that this was a choice based on feeling. He was attuned to what felt right for his way of being (see Chapter 12 in which Kent writes in more depth about his journey).

Carolyn recognises her fit with the approach in making her choice:

> Grounded theory was one I played around with. But phenomenology, I realised that's how I have always thought, ever since I was a child. I've always thought about peeling off the onion layers. So, it came to me very naturally.

Carolyn had heard phenomenology and knew it was "her tune." She already understood that meanings lay hidden. Peeling back, again and again aligned naturally with her thinking.

Jo pondered on how she might help someone else understand the "fit":

> If I were to guide someone new to this, I think I would start with Gadamer's ideas of horizons. What are my horizons? How do I interpret and how do you know that? How do I articulate my story, the way that I think of my story, the way that I think of who I am, where does that come from? And starting to have a realisation of the totality and the depth of that, that we never normally ever think of.

Jo articulates the big "what" and "how" questions of hermeneutic phenomenology that she herself wrestled with along the way. She points to the quest to see the "whole" and then to recognise the depth within. It is about being willing to examine and re-examine "self," owning the interpretive nature of all that one understands. It is to attune to the world in a new way, thinking through probing questions.

## Attuning to pre-understandings

It is our custom to do a pre-understandings interview as a beginning point in the interpretive journey of a thesis. Carolyn remembers hers:

> Looking back on my pre-understandings interview, I think even at that time I had an inkling that this research was going to lead into very deep water. Probably deeper than I even imagined. And that's exactly what it did.

Carolyn's research explored the experience of burnout for case-loading midwives. In speaking-out her own experience of being on call around the clock, Carolyn attuned to the depths of feeling some of her own stories revealed. In sensing her own deep waters, she began to feel a mood of darkness that was later revealed by her participants.

Kent also talks of his pre-understandings interview:

> I remember almost an intuitive sense of a story unfolding. Within me, some parts were known to me, but other parts weren't. And they somehow came out. When I've reviewed the transcript, I'm going: "Wow did I say that? Hmm.

That's interesting. I didn't know that". So, in the moment there was a feeling of something occurring and clearly it was coming out of my mouth, not pre thought and then not even remembered until I re read it.

Kent describes a flow of words and stories that "came out." He was caught up in something not pre-thought; a feeling, a mood. It is as though something was released and free to flow-forth. On reading the transcript, he found parts he had no memory of saying. There is a sense of him being lost in the telling, immersed in the experience itself; attuned to its mood.

Jo, near the end of her research, reminded us that the pre-understandings interview is simply the beginning of an ongoing process of openness:

> My pre-understandings interview was the beginning of formally pulling apart my understandings Why did I come to this? How do I see it? And realising that, that needs to be a constant process of reflection. I think within the realisation of all those influences, therein lies the pathway to openness.

For Jo, to pull apart what one already knows is to be attuned to the notion that there are always more questions, always a layering that awaits peeling back. One cannot simply say "I am open." Rather one talks about always-being-open, an active pursuit of recognising how one's own understanding has been shaped, and how another person might understand in a different way. Perhaps the mood is one of humility, or a sense there is yet more, of a resoluteness to keep questioning. It is a mood that keeps questions in play.

## Attuning to methodology

When participants began interviewing, they took on being-phenomenological:

> When I was doing my grounded theory interviews, I had a clipboard on my knee with questions. I can remember getting towards the end saying: "now have we got through all our questions, oh no, hang on I haven't asked this." This time, doing phenomenology, I didn't have a clipboard on my knee at all. The interview was what it was. In the moment and of that moment. It felt like an experience of being rather than an experience of putting a task out there. It really felt different. Whereas the grounded theory interviews were about answering the questions, in this phenomenological experience the participants said what they wanted and needed to say. They said things that they didn't know they were going to say. (*Kent*)

To be attuned to the phenomenological way is to let go of pre-made questions. It is to trust that the stories will flow one from another. It is to be attuned to the emerging insights, gently drawing them forth in the moment. In such a mood of openness, the participant hears themselves saying things that they had no idea would come forth. There is releasement beyond anticipation. That is, the conversation emerges in a way that takes both the teller and the listener by surprise. Sometimes that comes in unexpected tears, or laughter, or a story remembered from long, long ago.

## Growing openness

Jo's research was on the meaning of thriving in an Accident and Emergency Department. Writing her proposal involved much pre-reading on the nature of thriving. She talks of how her first interview challenged her openness:

> My first interview surprised me. I went in with an assumption that most of our thriving was about connection and meeting a purpose. My first participant was a guy and his meaning and purpose was around fixing things. He loved to fix things. As he talked about it, I thought well you know that's so true, that is a really cool part of what we do. It made me purposefully be more open. And I to be more aware of my own assumptions going in.

It is one thing to declare one is "open." As Jo found, it is only when one is surprised by the meanings expressed by another person that one sees afresh one's own assumptions. As Jo opened her thinking, she also saw how fixing things made her feel good about her own practice. She had her first lesson in learning to attune to what surprised or challenged her previous assumptions.

## Attuning to hidden emotions

Carolyn, in her research on burnout, found herself drawn into emotional depths which she needed to sensitively attune to:

> Doing the interviews was really intense. Lots of tears. Lots of anger. And lots of terrible self-recognition of how bad it had been for them, not even recognising up until that point because they'd so normalised it and because it was hidden. They thought it was like pre-menopausal symptoms when it was actually burnout. Like one participant's said: "I'm so good now. I haven't thought about suicide for about two months". Some didn't want to go there. And some couldn't go there. Because they would say: "Oh I can't remember". So, I'd say "Did you have days when you thought you might be depressed?" "Oh, oh no but I do remember staying in pyjamas all day". And then I'd say "oh" and then "I remember, oh god". And then change the topic. So, there was a little bit of working it out as I went.

It is one thing to reveal that which lies hidden. It is another to respect the participants' readiness to face the reality of their situation. Carolyn attuned both to the cues that pointed to burnout and the withdrawal of the participants who did not want to see how burnt-out they had become. As researcher, she was also a caring colleague. Maybe if she could help these midwives' see their behaviour as "telling" they could better attune to their own situation. The hiddenness of burnout was its danger. Revealing the hidden called forth an ethical attunement within the tension of "do no harm" yet "stop the escalating danger."

## Attuning to poetic meaning

Carolyn goes on to describe how poetic writing became part of her way of attuning:

> I started to think, yes this is so much bigger and much more damaging than what I ever imagined it because it was so hidden. The poems just slowly started to come. They were of 'I thought this is what burnout was, but it wasn't'. I'd go to the next interview and I'd find out another layer to it, something else there that was under the surface, Then I would re write the next bit of this as the next thing that had come up.

Listening, attuning to what was being said and not-said, beginning to peel back to reveal that which lay hidden was something Carolyn found herself doing after each interview by means of letting-a-poem-come. She would start by writing "I thought it was x but it was y." Here is one of those poems:

> I thought burnout was made of fear
> but it was made of
> uninvited, unexpected
> tightly held tears
> that suddenly seep
> in an overflow
> of sorrow.
> That even years later
> still cannot wash away
> those barbwire memories
> of the pain
> that comes from
> the death of dreams.
> (Young et al., 2011)

## Attuning as interpreting

Like Carolyn, Kent talks about the ongoing listening to the audio-recording of the participants stories:

> I listened as well. There were times if I came to something and I go "oh I like this" I would find that and listen to it just to see if the tonality was there. It was "this feels like something. I like this". If we think about mood, is this being something I've been pulled into or I've seen that is meaningful or is this the mood that I happen to be in today? Is this a particular participant that I happen to like? Or I maybe know more.

It is one thing to feel a mood; it is another thing to make sense of what lies behind the mood. Kent shows that to be attuned is to question, to ponder, to challenge one's own thinking. Attunement does not mean one necessarily knows. Rather it points towards that which is still to be known. Wrestling with the question of what provoked or lies underneath mood can yield rich insight.

## Writing as attunement

Jo recognised a habit of needing to know before she started to write and having to learn to simply start writing:

> It is absolutely true that the way is to write. I keep resisting it. I keep resisting. Let me read a little bit more and then it will come to me. Yet once I start writing, then that takes me down different pathways. It is my freedom, yet it's not a complete freedom that I let happen. I write and then go back and look. I look and think, and then give it the space and the freedom. It's a mixture of playing with writing and reading. My reading has been, has become my dialogue. In reading I dialogue with Heidegger and with Gadamer and van Manen. (Jo)

The phenomenological way is to start to write even amidst not knowing where the writing will lead (such as described by Polly in Chapter 3, when the use of poetry called to her). It is to simply trust that the writing itself will find the pathway that leads to insight. Such writing is about handing oneself over to being attuned, phrase by phrase, word by word. A freedom emerges but not a complete freedom. Writing still demands a reader (which begins with self). Reading expects insights. Insights are fed by reading. And thus, the play of reading-writing-thinking circles on, always attuned to the quest. Within such writing is the call to be open, to wonder afresh, to follow the possibilities that emerge in our mooded-thinking.

## Reading as attunement

Kent describes how he has learnt to read in an attuned way:

> What that meant to me was then the search for literature could go to non-traditional places. I felt as though I had permission to spend time around that literature from anywhere and everywhere. As long as there was able to be an argument in the connection in terms of the flow to my story.

Kent embraced the phenomenological freedom of letting writing from "anywhere" catch his attention. Driving this was his attunement to his developing insight and argument. While some reading comes prior to the research, there is an ongoing quest to read towards the gathering sense of story that emerges from interpreting the data. Without conscious thinking, one attunes to a new reading, quickly discerning if one will read on or discard. Attunement finds the threads that connect with a mood of resonance, a glimpse of possibilities, a stirring up of wonder.

## Light bulb

Jo remembers a light bulb moment that happened amidst a Heidegger reading group of which we were a part:

> Reading Question Concerning Technology (Heidegger 1992) was a bit of a light bulb experience. I think that part of medicine that I really struggle with is what seems to be a move to 'paint by numbers' medicine. I can see some of the usefulness of it. But it feels like it takes away the art that I feel like I identify with. And that paper was a light bulb going on, saying 'this is why, this is what that's really about'. It was an aha moment both in kind of seeing the way that Heidegger was writing and what he was meaning and also understanding my own dilemma within the clinical space.

Jo was not reading Heidegger for the sake of understanding his work. Rather she was pursuing her thinking on the nature of "thriving" in an Accident and Emergency Department. When she came to "see" the technological mechanisms inherent in clinical practice, she saw the danger wherein humanity gets pushed aside. Her attunement revealed itself in excited discussion. She began to play with ideas, making connections, discerning afresh that "thriving" was her quest to privilege humanity. It was as though her attunement heard the notes that now made a tune she recognised deep within her spirit.

## Attuning within the darkness of chaos

To linger deep within attunement is to sometimes find oneself lost:

> I think in writing the chapters I had been quite chaotic. It's almost as if the chaos is a way of freeing oneself of any attachment to anything. I had been quite chaotic in my gathering. But at the same time there were things that just kept jumping out at me. Like 'holding' was one. It just kept jumping out, but it was everywhere. I thought 'what am I going to do with this? Is this a whole chapter or is it in every chapter?' It feels an intuitive process. It took so long. I can see in my journals I'd get kind of 'I've got to get this, got to pin down the structure' and I'd scribble away and then it would just be 'oh no that's not it'. I was getting lost in Heidegger; it's very easy to get lost in Heidegger. There was one time when I was in the darkest place of the whole journey. I got really, really sick. For two weeks I didn't touch a thing. Something in me, I think, was trying to figure it out. But suddenly it was there. It did, it just suddenly came. It's almost like I had to go into Heidegger in those depths to get something to understand something. (*Margot*)

Margot was researching her own experience of being a teacher of psychotherapy students. Colleagues and ex-students interviewed her drawing from her stories of her experience of teaching. Thus, she was deeply attuned to her research, so much so that in the writing, chaos emerged. Reading Heidegger gifted her with deep thinking. As she gathered her thoughts together through journal writing, she struggled with teasing out the threads of the argument. Were they warp threads that went through the whole chapter, or weft threads that were to be dealt with in one place? It was following two weeks of being so sick she could not work on her thesis that the key insight "came." She recognised that it needed all the chaotically colourful tangled threads to enable the picture to emerge. In her non-thinking attunement, she "knew" all-at-once. Such knowing could never be achieved by a step-by-step rational method. It was rather a mammoth struggle from which the gem of understanding emerged (see Chapter 8 for more of Margot's journey).

## Emerging insights

> Writing should be easier than it is, and more fun. In trying to make it so, somehow, we all – teachers, students, beginning writers – got off track and made it, I think, more difficult instead. We started talking about errors and how to stay away from them; about the 'rules' of the game – watching or comma faults, making sure we had an 'introduction' and a 'body' and a 'conclusion', devising 'outlines,' living in fear we would violate the rules of 'unity' and 'coherence.'
>
> (Horton, 1982, 1)

All of us came to hermeneutic phenomenological research through the pathway of academia where we were indoctrinated into rules that bred disciplined ways of planning, enacting, thinking and writing. These rules have, and will continue to serve us well, yet perhaps the first step for the researcher new to hermeneutic phenomenological research is to set aside such cognitive, prescribed ways. It is rather to embrace a freedom that returns to primordial, ontological ways of being human.

Heidegger (2001, 140) brought a challenge to questions of research which *"intrude in the manner of precalculation and control"* or of *dealing with assumed universal representations which he named "concepts"* (141). Rather he brought us back to what it means to be human within our everyday lived experience, our ontological disposition [*Befindlichkeit*]. Dasein, our being-there, being-open (Sheehan, 2001) means that our attunement is always within a context of place, people, and whatever else constitutes our world in that situation. In other words, we "attune" to how we are in the moment with all the threads that weave together to make that moment uniquely itself. Freeman offers an overview of Heidegger's basic structures of human existence, otherwise known as existentialia:

> Dasein is understood … in terms of existentialia: necessary and basic structures of human existence[which] are the ontological structures that constitute the way humans exist in the world. The basic existentialia are attunement

[*Befindlichkeit*], understanding [*Verstehen*], discourse [*Rede*] (and fallenness [*Verfallenheit*]).

(Freeman, 2014, 448)

One cannot write about "attuning-to" without also talking what helps us make sense of the mood, and the understanding that emerges, spoken into words that may (or may not) be understood by others. It is important to always remember that one of Heidegger's existentialia is fallenness. In fallenness, Dasein is: "'*lost in the publicness of the They' [others with whom we share our social words]: it mostly continues to act and think in traditional ways*" (Inwood, 2000, 66–67) (also discussed by Lesley Kay in Chapter 5 and Jean in Chapter 11). This means that, even though one may attune, in language which seeks to understand, one is likely to be drawn back into the taken-for-granted interpretations of "the They." For example, the participant says, with a tremble in her voice, "I might have to pull out of my doctorate." Already we fall into thinking "she is finding it too hard; she can't afford the fees; her life is too busy." With sensitive attunement the authentic interpretation of what underlies her sentiment maybe something we never imagined.

Perhaps the key starting point is to recognise that we can be no other way than attuned (Heidegger 1962), yet, as Horton (1982) recognised in her book on writing, many of us have had our primordial way of being schooled out of us. The participants in this research felt the already-thereness of phenomenological ways in their experience of "being me." They delighted in the freedom to set aside rules, methods and adherence-to and instead tune-in to their feelings, their mood, their sense of grasping something that mattered. At the same time, they needed to unlearn some entrenched behaviours of following a plan, looking for facts, predetermining the argument before writing. They had to "become" phenomenological.

This *"becoming"* was to return to the wonder of childhood where one is arrested by the beauty of the butterfly and wonder how it emerged from its chrysalis (with a similar metaphor identified in Jean's PhD – see Chapter 11). It is to put aside (for a time) the rules of academic writing where nothing can be written without an associated reference. It is to break free of what one has been schooled "ought" to be done, in a neat, orderly, boring manner. It is rather to dance to the music one half-hears that stirs one into drawing closer. Creativity, excitement, getting-lost, exploring untrodden pathways, finding treasures hidden amidst the taken-for-grantedness; this is the uncharted way of hermeneutic phenomenology.

Who we are matters in this mode of research. Everything we already know and understand, and the very words that hold such meanings, has arisen through our own life journey (Gadamer, 1982). As Gadamer writes: "*The important thing is to be aware of one's own bias, so that the text may present itself in all its newness and thus be able to assert its own truth against one's own fore-meaning*" (238). He goes on: "*This recognition that all understanding inevitably involves some prejudices gives the hermeneutical problem its real thrust*" (239). This quest to be ongoingly open to the assumptions one brings as researcher protects us from simply assuming our mood is irrelevant to what we "should" be focused on. Instead, we ask: "what is it about this mood that disturbs/excites/bewilders me?" Beginning the research journey with a preunderstandings interview gives a benchmark of passion and insight, of excitement and concern, of clarity and confusion. Carolyn, for example, came to see she herself had some stories that reflected times of coming close to burnout. Openness, as Jo found, comes when a participant talks of something that is different from what one expected. Openness brings the questions that lead to understanding.

Attuning to the mood of wonder and openness to that which captures us and holds our thrall is something that needs "attention." Gendlin (1978–79) tells us: *"We may not know what the mood is about, we may not even be specifically aware of our mood"* (3). Academia has not schooled us in listening to our feelings as we read an article. Yet there have been some like Peshkin (1988) who recognised the importance of attuning to one's warm and cool spots when reading and responding to data. It is a different experience to go into an interview seeking to be attuned as opposed to following a list of pre-made questions. To be attuned in our hermeneutic phenomenological projects is to listen beyond what is said, to feel and respond to the emotions that are exposed, to know when to hold the silence, to recognise that one's own response will influence what gets told (or not) (Fiumara, 1990). We attune to the words that are said, how they are said, and the feelings they provoke in us. In other words, Heidegger's existentialia of attunement, discourse and understanding come together as Dasein, as being-there and being-open. All this is within the thrownness of the situation. A story emerges that neither expected to hear. One's own emotions startle and draw one into the profound nature of what is being revealed.

Researchers using other methodological approaches will still be impacted by the tears that come amidst the telling of a story. They will still pick up a transcript with delight as they remember it was a great interview. They will wander off from their task of writing feeling stuck. To be human is to always be attuned, for moods are always with us. However, it is the hermeneutic phenomenological researcher who learns to pay attention to those moods, to ponder them, to let wondering take them on a journey of coming to "see." They will come to see that attunement is their guide to "the way."

When it comes to the discourse of writing down the emerging understanding, the hermeneutic phenomenological writer holds open the freedom to attune to the saying-that-comes while at the same time questioning what is being said. The writing itself throws them into trying to grasp that which at the same time eludes. Out of the chaos emerges a moment of startling clarity. The understanding has come because the person has attuned to all that "spoke" and questioned how it came to be so. They re-read the paragraph written yesterday with a sense that there is something here worthy of being said. Something important has been revealed. How do they know that? They simply know in a bodily kind of way. They share a particular story in a large lecture theatre full of people. In the reading, a deep silence "comes." It has "touched." The story has spoken. The interpretation that follows gets the nod: "Yes. That is how it is. Now I understand what I somehow already knew." Hermeneutic phenomenology gifts in ways beyond the researcher's words. It speaks to the mood of another in a way that impacts their being. It is never finished. The wondering lives on.

> *And so we say:*
>
> Attuning-to is the beginning place, the ongoing quest and the way to light-bulb moments.
> It is to listen attentively without trying to 'hear'.
> It is to let the experience of being-there infuse wonder.
> It is be alert to the familiarity of everyday.
> Everything is waiting for you.
> Savour the moment. Be open to its gifts.

## Notes

1. Dreyfus referred to mood or attunement as how one is faring is the mood; e.g. how one is faring in our projects, or how one is faring in a meeting – not so much individual but an overall "feel" of the meeting. See Dreyfus, H.L. 1991. *Being-in-the-world: A commentary on Heidegger's Being and Time,* division I. Cambridge, MA: MIT Press.
2. Explore more about crafting stories in Crowther, S., P. Ironside, D. Spence, and L. Smythe. 2017. "Crafting stories in hermeneutic phenomenology research: A methodological device." *Qualitative Health Research* 27 (6): 826–835. doi: 10.1177/1049732316656161.
3. Existentialia, is an entity whose Being is only present-at-hand and which are understood ontically, whereas existence refers to entities whose Being is an issue for Dasein, who are understood as ontological. Existentiale, the plural of existentialia, are Dasein's characteristics revealed to the phenomenologist through analysis of existence.

## References

Fiumara, G.C. 1990. *Midwifery and philosophy. The other side of language: A philosophy of listening.* New York, NY: Routledge.

Freeman, L. 2014. "Toward a phenomenology of mood." *Southern Journal of Philosophy* 52 (4): 445. https://ezproxy.aut.ac.nz/login?url=https://search.ebscohost.com/login.aspx?direct=true&db=edb&AN=103265162&site=eds-live.

Gadamer, H.G. 1982. *Truth and method.* New York, NY: Crossroad.

Gadamer, H.G. 2006a. "Artworks in word and image: 'So true, so full of being!' (Goethe) (1992)." *Theory, Culture and Society* 23 (1): 57–83. https://doi.org/10.1177/0263276406063229. https://ezproxy.aut.ac.nz/login?url=https://search.ebscohost.com/login.aspx?direct=true&db=edselc&AN=edselc.2-52.0-33644928325&site=eds-live.

Gadamer, H.-G. 2006b. "Language and understanding(1970)." *Theory, Culture & Society* 23 (1): 13–27. https://doi.org/10.1177/0263276406063226. http://tcs.sagepub.com/content/23/1/13.abstract.

Gelven, M. 1970. *A commentary of Heidegger's Being and Time.* New York: Harper Torchbooks.

Gendlin, E. 1978–79. "Befindlichkeit: Heidegger and the philosophy of psychology." *Review of Existential Psychology & Psychiatry: Heidegger and Psychology* XVI (I): 2 & 3.

Heidegger, M. 1962. *Being and Time*. Translated by J. Macquarrie and E. Robinson. Oxford, UK: Blackwell Publishers Ltd. 1927.

—. 1975. "The Thing." In *Poetry, language, thought*, 163–186. New York, NY: Harper Row.

—. 1992. "Question Concerning Technology." In *Basic writings*, edited by D.F. Krell, 307–341. New York: HarperCollins.

Heidegger, M. 1968. *What is called thinking?* Translated by J.G. Gray. New York, NY: Harper Row.

—. 2001. *Zollikon seminars*. Translated by F. Mayr and R. Askay and edited by M. Boss. Evanston, IL: Northwestern University Press. 1987.

Horton, S. 1982. *Thinking through writing*. Baltimore, MD: Johns Hopkins University Press.

Inwood, M.J., 2000. *Heidegger: A very short introduction* (Vol. 25). Oxford: Oxford Paperbacks.

Kisiel, T. 2002. *Heidegger's way of thought: Critical and interpretive signposts*. New York, NY: Continuum.

Peshkin, A. 1988. "On search of subjectivity – One's own." *Educational Researcher* (October): 7–21.

Sheehan, T. 2001. "A Paradigm shift in Heidegger research." *Continental Philosophy Review* XXXII (2): 1–20. https://doi.org/10.1023/A:1017568025461.

Smythe, E., and D. Spence. 2019. "Reading Heidegger." *Nursing Philosophy: An International Journal for Healthcare Professionals*: e12271–e12271. https://doi.org/10.1111/nup.12271. http://ezproxy.aut.ac.nz/login?url=http://search.ebscohost.com/login.aspx?direct=true&db=cmedm&AN=31314178&site=eds-live.

Smythe, E., and D. Spence. 2020. "Heideggerian phenomenological hermeneutics: Working with the data." *Nursing Philosophy*. https://doi.org/10.1111/nup.12308. https://ezproxy.aut.ac.nz/login?url=https://search.ebscohost.com/login.aspx?direct=true&db=edselc&AN=edselc.2-52.0-85087290659&site=eds-live.

van Manen, M. 1990. *Researching lived experience*. Ontario: The University of Western Ontario.

van Manen, M. 2014. *Phenomenology of practice*. Walnut Creek, CA: Left Coast Press.

Whyte, D. 2007. *River flow*. Langley, Washington: Many Rivers Press.

Young, C.M., E. Smythe, and J. McAra-Couper. 2011. *The experience of burnout in case loading midwives: An interpretive phenomenological study: A thesis presented in fulfilment of the requirements for the degree of Doctor of Philosophy, 2011*, School of Health Sciences, Auckland University of Technology.

# 3 Using poetry to illuminate the lived accounts of Juvenile Dermatomyositis in children and young people

*Polly Livermore*

## Abstract

This chapter describes a study to capture children and young people's experience of a rare, chronic, life threatening condition called Juvenile Dermatomyositis (JDM). The study interviewed children and young people between the ages of 8 and 19 years of age, all with a diagnosis of JDM in one London Tertiary Hospital. After the first few interviews, but before the beginnings of analysis, whilst re-reading, reflecting and ruminating, the words of my participants were crafted into research poems. In this chapter, I describe the process I took in viewing the *thrownness* of JDM as transforming ones *Being-in-the-world*, via poetry offerings to provide an in-depth, powerful representation of this condition.

## Introduction

The beauty of hermeneutic phenomenology is that it offers the ability to capture rich lived experiences, and to interpret and understand the effects of living with a chronic, rare health condition. This understanding is vital for health care workers, to equip us with in-depth knowledge to consider all aspects of ill health on an individual. When that individual is a child or young person, that understanding is even more important as it allows an insight into their daily world; an insight which they might not always be able to express as clearly as those with adult vocabulary and life experience. In the following sections, I describe the nature, prevalence and impact of Juvenile Dermatomyositis (JDM), the complexities of actually "doing" a hermeneutic phenomenology study and how I achieved the "phenomenological nod." I draw on Heidegger's concept of *Being-in-the-world* to illuminate their psychosocial needs and *thrownness* to illustrate the complexities of capturing lived experience from paediatric patients.

## Juvenile Dermatomyositis

JDM is a rare, autoimmune disease of childhood that has no cure and risk of mortality. Beginning with typical skin rashes (particularly prominent on the face, elbows, knuckles and knees) and leading to progressive proximal muscle weakness, JDM can also affect many of the internal organs, especially if left untreated (Feldman et al., 2008; Kim et al., 2017). JDM has an annual incidence in the

DOI: 10.4324/9781003081661-3

United Kingdom of between 0.8 and 4.1 per million children per year, mean age of onset of seven years and a male-to-female ratio of 1:5 (Symmons, Sills and Davis, 1995; Batthish and Feldman, 2011). Diagnostic criteria are historically defined by Bohan and Peter (1975a, 1975b) as the presence of one of the defined characteristic rashes, combined with three of either: symmetrical proximal muscle weakness, raised serum muscle enzymes, abnormal findings on muscle biopsy and electromyography (EMG) (Feldman et al., 2008; Wedderburn and Rider, 2009).

JDM can occur rapidly or insidiously, with children and young people struggling to climb the stairs after a day at school or being unable to stand up from sitting on the floor. Without early diagnosis and initiation of treatment, children and young people may become bedbound, unable to sit up or roll over and for some, they may even require nutritional support through feeding tubes (Batthish and Feldman, 2011; Ernste and Reed, 2014). In severe cases, this debilitating condition involves children and young people requiring multiple hospitalisations, experiencing extreme muscle pain, requiring daily physiotherapy and cytotoxic (cell-killing) medications to gain symptom control, and as a result, they may miss months of schooling (Lowry and Pilkington, 2009; Deakin et al., 2018). Many children and young people continue to have active disease and irreversible damage from their disease and/or treatment into adulthood (Ravelli et al., 2010). Current research into JDM is focused upon identifying biomarkers in the blood which may predict disease course or seeking to trial new therapies, with research examining psychosocial needs being sparse. Furthermore, research attempting to present psychosocial needs (pertaining to both psychological and social) have predominantly asked parents and caregivers what is it like for a child or young person to live with JDM (Apaz et al., 2009; Kountz-Edwards et al., 2017), ultimately excluding the voices of those who actually experience this disease.

## Why I adopted Hermeneutic Phenomenology

My study embraced the methodology of hermeneutic phenomenology to describe, understand and interpret experience from those experiencing JDM (McConnell-Henry, Chapman, and Francis, 2009; Smythe, 2011; Tuohy et al., 2013). As there had been no studies into young people's experience of this condition, I felt this approach would enable me to help illuminate the reality for them, to live with and experience this condition.

Martin Heidegger (1889–1976), famous for his hermeneutic phenomenology approach, which moved from description to interpretation and deriving meaning from *Being-in-the-world* (McConnell-Henry, Chapman and Francis, 2009). The situated meaning of a human, or *Dasein* as Heidegger termed it, *Being-in-the-world*, is being capable of wondering about one's own existence (MacKey, 2005). *Being-in-the-world* refers to the way human beings are involved in the world, constructed from our own backgrounds and experiences. Consequently, pre-understanding is not something a person can step outside of because nothing can be encountered without reference to a person's background understanding (Laverty, 2017). Moreover, I believe the experience of a child's illness cannot be told through the eyes of a parent or caregiver but only be truly told by the one who experiences it. This was an essential element to my study, to ask the children and young people themselves about their *Being-in-the-world* whilst living with JDM.

## Becoming reflexive

Hermeneutic phenomenology embraces the notion that the researcher's subjective personal knowledge, judgement and preunderstandings cannot be separated from their study (Walker, 2007). Being transparent about my background and journey to this research led to the question in my study; to foreground this process, I had a "pre-suppositions interview" (sometimes termed pre-understandings interview), a device promoted in hermeneutic phenomenology (Spence, 2016) (also discussed in depth in Chapter 2).

A senior hermeneutic phenomenologist at the University of Central Lancashire interviewed me in May 2017. I was questioned in depth about my prior experience of nursing children with JDM. Some of the preunderstandings that emerged from this reflective experience stemmed from my experience as a newly qualified staff nurse over 20 years ago from caring for 2 young children with JDM. These two children, despite being different genders, nationalities and from completely different social backgrounds, both had in common a shared affect. They both developed a loss of ability to communicate with those around them, becoming frightened and sad as they withdrew from daily interaction. I tried hard in my new nursing role to engage them in the world around them, and it would be the highlight of my day if I could get them to smile. Both these young children, unfortunately, passed away. Being newly qualified, I had a strong desire to provide the best nursing care possible, with a primary focus on helping people recover from illness. I had not experienced death in a patient that I was caring for before and found that my role in this situation changed. I was not the parent but still wanted to grieve the loss of their young lives.

Since this time, I have nursed many other children and young people with JDM and observed a range of coping mechanisms utilised by young people. Due to the chronic nature of this condition, the children and their families are frequently reviewed in the hospital over many years, leading to close relationships developing with their health teams. At certain times, for example, at disease flares, I became attuned to spotting changes in their affect, and as my own confidence, experience and knowledge has continued to grow, I have felt that we could be better at supporting these patients to live with their condition. This reflective engagement provided an insight into my own preunderstandings and helped illustrate how these had brought me to this research area and, subsequently, this present study.

## Being creative

In hermeneutic phenomenology, the interview serves a very specific purpose; a vehicle to develop a conversational relationship with the participant about the meaning of an experience and allowing participants to share their stories in their own words (Ajjawi and Higgs, 2007). However, there is very little research about conducting phenomenological interviews with children and young people. Research with children is different to research with adults for a number of important reasons (Gallacher and Gallagher, 2008; Clark et al., 2014):

- There is a power imbalance between adult researchers and child participants.
- Children may lack the language to explain their point of view.
- Children are often protected by gatekeepers.
- They may need "tools" and artefacts to tell their stories.
- Adults often think they know what is important to children and young people without the need to ask them.

The phenomenological interview is inherently a "conversation" (Wise, 2002), yet, conversations with children can be difficult for the above reasons. As Ford et al. (2017) explain, if children have to rely solely on the use of words, it can be difficult for them to articulate their experiences. Some studies have alluded to the difficulties of carrying out open-ended phenomenological interviews with children and young people (Wise, 2002; Kostenius and Öhrling, 2009; Shi, 2013; Livermore, Eleftheriou and Wedderburn 2016). These authors and others have discussed a variety of activities to encourage children to talk freely. I realised I needed to be creative in my approaches.

A phenomenological study of children's experiences relies upon data given through a language, and so it would seem appropriate to include creative methods, such as children's drawings, singing or playing, as expressed in their own language (Danaher and Briod, 2012). By adding a creative method into the interview, some of the limitations of interviewing children, such as having a limited vocabulary compared to adults (Punch, 2002), can be overcome whilst still enabling them to tell their stories. In my study, I offered them a range of creative methods, including; body-mapping (also used in Helen and Elizabeth's work – Chapter 7), an electronic timeline and comic book drawing. I was also aware that not all young people like creative methods and may prefer to talk about their experiences in a face-to-face interview (Carter and Ford, 2013). Multiple methods were therefore offered to aid them to share their experience.

## Interview challenges

This study was undertaken as part of a much larger National Institute of Health Research (NIHR) funded Clinical Doctoral Research Fellowship (CDRF, Fellowship number ICA-CDRF-2016-02-032) to obtain a Doctor of Philosophy (Ph.D.), in the summer of 2017 in a Tertiary hospital in London. Following ethical approval,[1] including specific permission to use participant words in dissemination; 15 children and young people were recruited. Children and young people were included if they were between the ages of 8 and 19 years of age, had a diagnosis of JDM and assented/consented with parental informed consent. I offered a choice of interview location, either whilst at an appointment at the hospital or at a later date in their own home. Two interviews had mothers present in the room, and where they joined in the conversation, this was clearly documented throughout.

The majority preferred to just talk rather than be creative, and on reflection, these interviews involved fewer questions and were longer in duration. It was apparent as the study progressed that creative methods were more appealing to the youngest participants. However, these methods were not without challenges. For example, the electronic timeline, whilst being enjoyed by the young child had turned into a hindrance to free speech as the desire to get facts correctly typed into the electronic app and spelt correctly took much time. The comic book drawing had also gone off on a tangent as the young child drew rainbows and flowers, with a limited verbal discussion about the experiences of JDM. From these points, I add a caution to other phenomenological researchers that whilst these methods sound "easy" on paper, in practice, they may be anything but easy. The parental perspective also offered a further "challenge," whilst it was ethical to have their involvement if they (and the participant) so wished, it was hard to disentangle the parental voice from the child/young person. I was left questioning whether parents had led their child or young person or whether their adult comments had changed the direction of the conversation. Ultimately, I decided to weave their voices throughout the transcripts where possible. One could question whether this is an appropriate thing to do, especially as I acknowledged at the beginning that parents cannot share the depth of the experience of JDM as the child themselves, but involving the parents in paediatric care is always a challenge and often results in a shared perspective (Smith, Swallow and Coyne, 2015).

## Dwelling with the data

After the first few interviews, before analysis had even been contemplated, I found there were certain words which kept playing on repeat. One interview with a young girl had been particularly moving. The 90-minute interview had been charged with emotion, with the participant, mother and myself all in tears. The words used during this interview would return to me at unexpected times; when brushing my teeth or tucking my children up into bed at night. Finally, as I was walking to a meeting one day, I felt I had no choice but to stop and sit on a bench, with a notebook ready to capture the flyaway thoughts which were tumbling around inside my head. The result was a poem, a poem of her words stuck together to illustrate her experience in only a few lines of text. The end result was:

*Tomato Face*

"Tomato face" they called me,
Come on guys, can't you see,
My face looks more like a "baboons bum",
Bright red, swollen, horrible, really not fun,

You can't hide your face, can you?
If your arms get fat, you cover them up, that's what you do,
"Don't worry" the doctors say,
"We're not worried that you're a little redder today",
But the fear is that after a little, comes a lot,
And that my JDM just won't stop.
(Livermore, Wedderburn and Gibson, 2020, 22)

The poem was crafted within a few minutes as if someone else had taken over. I had not written poetry since school, many, many years previously, but upon completion, it was clear that the poem succinctly encapsulated what this teenager had experienced.

Hermeneutic phenomenology challenges the researcher to show the experience without value judgements or prejudice, and despite not setting out to create poetry, this final offering did just that. This poem helped to make accessible Heidegger's notion of *thrownness*. Heidegger uses the term *Dasein* to depict how as human beings, we always already exist in a world of meaning – a *"being-there"* in an interconnected totality where our understanding is shaped by the culture and society of the world we inhabit. He also considers how Dasein is always being *thrown* into different situations, often with no volition (a Heideggerian term also considered by Lesley Dibley in Chapter 6). For the children and young people in this study, they are *thrown* into the world of JDM, of hospitals, of treatments, of looking different, of feeling different. For this teenage girl, in her new day-to-day world of living with JDM, she thinks differently as she pre-empts the thoughts of others. Her *thrownness* informs her way of *Being-in-the-world*, beyond her control and in a particular way. The crafted poetry enabled me to powerfully illuminate the *thrownness* experienced, which would have been hard to find amongst pages of the transcript.

However, at this point, I began to question myself to see if what I had done was okay, allowed even. It was with great delight that I found a huge evidence base for what I had just created.

## From prose to poetics

There are three main ways poetry can be used in research, summarised by Faulkner (2009) as:

- Poems presented to research participants for critique;
- Poetry to present themes noted by the researcher;
- Poems created from research transcripts.

In my study, poems were created from research transcripts, as a powerful method of data presentation, prior to any structured and planned data analysis. I was delighted to find out that what I had just done had many names in the literature, including; "Research poems," "Poetic representation," "Poetic transcriptions" and

"Found poems." However, all of these have the same rules: the words can be juxtaposed from anywhere in the transcript, but in a way that does not change the essence (Glesne, 1997), and they should respect the participants' culture, their understanding and their lived experience (Clarke and Iphofen, 2006). After my first spontaneous experience, I went on to create further poems from some of the remaining transcripts. Whilst the poems use repetition, similes, imagery, pauses and rhyme (Öhlen, 2003), the words spoken are always those from the young people themselves.

Poetry played a crucial role in Heidegger's later thinking, and in his "Origins of the work of art" he contends that poetry has a place in human experience (Page, 2018). He perceived that poetry can uncover the *Being-in-the-world*, making visible that which was un-visible (Hofstager, 1988):

> The poem is now already no longer a bland text with some correspondingly flat 'meaning' attached to it; rather, this configuring of language is in itself a turbulence that tears us away somewhere. Not gradually; rather, we are torn away suddenly and abruptly right at the beginning.
>
> (Heidegger, 2014, 45)

Poetry also further mirrors the aim of hermeneutics attentiveness to language and to gain an understanding of texts (McCulliss, 2013) and that of phenomenology which is to be open to the experience as it is told. Poetry has the potential to transform the way we perform research and the ability to present our findings in a more captivating, evocative and insightful way (McCulliss, 2013). Poetry, therefore, fits perfectly with hermeneutic phenomenology and was a perfect medium to reveal the experience of JDM.

## Crafting the poems

Through my early beginning of just free writing a poem, I learnt that there is no one way to create research poems: instead, each poet reflects on the way they did it on that occasion (Glesne, 1997). Miller (2018), for example, describes the five steps they took:

1 Deep data immersion
2 Arranging words to create the poem
3 Critical reflection on the quality of each poem
4 Researcher reflexivity and member checking
5 Engagement and dissemination

Steps 1–3 make the process sound easy, however, in practice, I did not find them straightforward. Each interview had yielded numerous pages of the transcript which needed to be read, considered and reflected upon. This process took time. I looked for clear messages, strong emotion, repetitive phrases and especially an essence of that young person's personality, a snapshot of who they are with JDM.

Within some transcripts, the process was easier than in others and led to more than one poem being crafted, in others, it took me some time to find the poem. The poems were reflected upon and checked for trustworthiness by my research team to ensure I had not added words or taken the meaning out of context.

In all qualitative research, the researcher sifts through the data and presents it in a manner that is meaningful to them, and different exerts will always tell different stories (McCulliss, 2013). This process of moving text around and shaping it into poems for the audience is no different. To illustrate the trustworthy process undertaken, the following example is shown in the text below. The text is taken from one of the interviews, and the italic text illustrates the words that were lifted out to make the below poem entitled "Why me." This is only a snapshot, not all words are visible to protect patient confidentiality, however, this exert provides an example of the process:

It sometimes hurts here on both arms, especially when I go *to* physiotherapy or I exercise. Also, sometimes my throat feels *sore* when I'm upset. *It hurts* sometimes on both legs high up and my ankles, especially when I *walk*.

I sometimes feel upset when I start to get pain and sometimes, I get a headache. My tummy sometimes hurts, I think it's because I need the toilet. I get very hungry, they said it's the medicine. I think my medicines are too much. I have to have them all the time. They don't really help me, and some of them taste really bad.

I can talk to my mum if I'm in pain or sad, but sometimes *I don't wanna talk* and I just want to be quiet. I have a question for you? *Why me*, why did I all of a sudden fall sick?

The poem "Why me?" was shaped from this interview transcript:

*Why me?*

Why me?
It's so unfair,
Why me?
It hurts everywhere,
Why me?
It hurts to walk,
Why me?
I don't wanna talk,
Why me?
I miss my life before,
Why me?
My life before I got sore.

This interview had been particularly challenging. As the youngest participant of the study, with the newest diagnosis and as a current inpatient in a hospital, encouraging them to talk to me as a stranger was tricky. This participant had chosen to draw in the comic book to help tell their story without the need for eye contact.

Further poems from other participants then followed quickly. I found if I entwined details stated during the interview, such as their age, then this provided a more comprehensive picture for the reader, helping them to understand who owned the experience, such as:

Worry

You give me a name that I can't say,
But I have to explain what it is every day,
I am ten now, but I worry about how I will be,
What is my JDM doing to me?
It's not easy to see,
But I know it's there inside me.
(Livermore, Wedderburn and<br>Gibson, 2020, 24)

The power of using poems to convey children and young people's accounts was apparent when I presented a lecture at a predominantly medical conference. Prior to the meeting, I had a conversation with one of the medical professionals, who told me that he rarely spoke to children and young people in the clinic about their JDM. Children and young people often did not engage in the consultations, so it made more sense (and was timelier) to communicate to the parent. However, after my presentation, which began and ended with the "Worry" poem, the professional came to me to say he would be changing his practice and talking to all young people, regardless of how quiet or young they were. As I read out this poem during the conference, there was a silence, a stillness as if all were holding their breaths. After the presentation, healthcare professionals told me that I had caused a "ripple effect of goosebumps." This was a moment of elation as I truly understood what Smythe (2011) had been referring to as the "phenomenological nod," a moment of shared resonance aspired to by all hermeneutic phenomenologists.

## Resonance

Whilst researcher reflexivity was vital, the recommended "member checking" often prescribed in qualitative research – where data is returned to the participants to ensure words had not been taken out of context – was more of an ethical concern as I was anxious about whether this would cause distress to the children and young people. Any harm caused by research, such as the potential for children and young people to become upset when reading and reflecting on their thoughts of living with a chronic condition, should be avoided. This was very important to me and a position I had to defend on numerous occasions. However, in support of this stance, Crowther et al. (2017) highlights that returning the text or member checking is questionable in hermeneutic phenomenology because human understanding is evolving and therefore always open and on the way to constantly new revisions and interpretations.

However, on two occasions, I made a carefully considered decision to share the poems I had crafted. In both instances, the decision stemmed from a desire to help the individuals – not as a process of member checking. Their personal struggle with JDM was clearly evident during their interviews, and I felt the poetry could help them to share their thoughts with others if they so wished. In one instance, the poetry was first discussed with the young person's mother to gauge whether she thought it was a good idea and to prevent an undue upset. The mother agreed that the poem was exactly what she needed to help her know she was understood. On the other occasion, the poem was directly offered to the young person so they could share how one of their medications; methotrexate, made them feel. Methotrexate is a cytotoxic medication often used as a cancer treatment, but also for many autoimmune conditions and is known for causing sickness, even prior to taking the therapy (Mulligan et al., 2013; Livermore, 2014; Ferrara et al., 2018). This interview had yielded 26 pages of transcript from an interview that lasted over two hours, most of which was spent explaining how methotrexate had overshadowed years of living with JDM.

This is the poem constructed from this young person's words:

*Methotrexate*

You were ok in the start,
I was too naïve to pull it apart,
Chalky horrible, disgusting thing, sticking in my throat,
Hiding in my chocolate mousse, never going to eat that again! (make a note),
Can't swallow any tablets now, (unfortunately),
Dad doesn't get it, I know I'm 18, but it's not my fault, it's what you've done to me,
I don't want you to win,
Why can't I beat you? Take it on the chin,
Whole day sick with nerves, all day afflicted,
Mum went to such trouble to get the liquid,
Now I have guilt on top of the fear as I shake my head,
I don't want it I said!
I physically can't, it's more than I don't want to,
It's deeper, that's so true,
I want to say I can do it each week and that you don't scare me,
But you do.
I know it's a mental thing,
I haven't even taken you yet and I'm retching,
I'm scared, what happens if I'm sick in the night, off school again tomorrow,
Another meal regurgitated down to you, smell forever etched on my brain, this time, risotto,
A dream combination so they say,
You and Azathioprine,
Hip hip hooray,
Not in my dreams, that's for sure,
My parents don't understand,
I don't understand, it's really getting out of hand,
It's so difficult to explain,

Tablets, liquids, injections all the same,
I wanted you for my skin, is that vain?
If you make me feel worse on a daily basis then what's the point?
Why do I disappoint?
I try so hard, I psych myself up, but I can't do it,
I don't want you to win, not even a bit,
Why can't I beat you? I wish I knew,
If I can't beat you, will I ever get better? I wish I knew.

Trying to succinctly capture the depth of this young person's "battle" with methotrexate throughout pages of the transcript, was challenging. However, the poem enabled these messages to come across clearly in key phrases. Whilst experiencing sickness from methotrexate is common, it was the extent of nausea and vomiting affecting her daily life which needed to be acknowledged. This sickness is typically not recognised enough by medical health care professionals, who see the disease benefit and require young people to persevere without really understanding the full emotional consequences (Livermore, 2014; Livermore and Begum, 2021). This young person had repeated many times that others could not understand what this experience had been like, and thus, the gift of the poem provided the voice to share what they struggled to say. Here is the reply from the young person after reading the poem:

The poem is beautiful and really does show how I feel, thank you so much for taking the time to write it!

Later that day, I received:

My parents just read it and it made them both cry! It really is beautifully written! Mum wanted me to ask if she can share it on her JDM page on [her social media account]?

These comments illustrate the power behind poems. Whilst stripped away from all the buffering text, each word is there to carry meaning. Knowing that the poem had captured what this adolescent had been trying to say for so long, helping them share this with their parents, truly made the process worthwhile. The poem was shared on a closed JDM social media page, and the many responses highlighted the resonance that other young people (and their parents) felt when reading the poem. This medication poem highlights the *Being-in-the-world* for this young person as one which is constructed from uncertainty and fear on a daily basis due to being *thrown* into the world of JDM and its treatments.

## Trustworthiness

The purpose of hermeneutic phenomenology is not to hammer home a point or to provide a fixed truth but to reveal taken-for-granted meanings and let the text speak. The expert hermeneutic phenomenologist is aiming for the "phenomenological nod" when the stories stir emotions and provoke quiet, thoughtful reflection in others. This is also true of poetry, whereby emotions and passion are central features of poetic work (Darmer, 2006).

The findings presented are always simply the impressions gained, an offering of thinking to engage others in their own thinking (Smythe et al., 2008) and thus open to further interpretation. Crafting short poems from reams of transcripts also carries the risk of bias. A different researcher may well have used different texts to end up with a different final poem (Prendergast, 2006). I was in charge of selecting the text to become the poem, and this in itself alters the interpretation of the data (Glesne, 1997). However, this is also true of hermeneutic phenomenology, in which it is "my experience" of what the data is telling me (Smythe, 2011). There is no single correct interpretation as we are constantly open to new information (McCulliss, 2013), opening to new horizons of understanding. Methods to help us uphold rigour and trustworthiness are, however, essential. In my study, this was achieved through transparency in how the poems were crafted, an audit trail of methodological decisions and reflexivity.

## Finding the phenomena

Whilst the focus of this chapter is on the creation of the poetry from the transcripts, it seemed appropriate to conclude with a summary of what happened after the poetry, with the rest of the data and the phenomena of JDM.

Whilst attending an enlightening hermeneutic phenomenology course in 2017, I had been moved by listening to "stories" crafted from interview transcripts from midwives and wanted to use this approach on my research data. I followed the process of how to "craft" or "derive" narratives from transcripts described by Caelli (2001), my own interpretation of these steps is illustrated in Table 3.1.

*Table 3.1* The process of how to derive narratives from transcripts

|   | Task |
| --- | --- |
| 1 | Reading and re reading whole interview many times |
| 2 | Highlighting the first level extra text which can come out, for example, or listening noises where not important, and "umms" and "huh" which are extra, remove this |
| 3 | Identify sections that wander away from phenomena, are superfluous, for example, when discussing the weather or what they had for lunch or do not make good grammatical English and remove |
| 4 | Interviewer questions deleted or marked for clarification |
| 5 | Add conjoining words to make it readable, but keeping participant words wherever possible |
| 6 | Craft into chronological story, in a way that "shows" what the researcher is noticing and interpreting whilst working with the data and keeping it true to original meaning |
| 7 | With comments added to show initial thoughts on themes of each paragraph of crafted story |
| 8 | Return to participants for "member checking" |

This crafting process has been further described by Crowther et al. (2017). Whilst this was a flexible and intuitive process, it highlighted the challenges of adopting an unbounded approach whilst needing to demonstrate rigour – the steps taken during analysis were documented, reviewed and kept securely to provide a clear audit trail.

The only step not undertaken as suggested by Caelli (2001) was the final stage of returning the end text to the participant for "member checking," for the reasons explained earlier.[2]

## Being-on-the-JDM-rollercoaster

The process, as discussed by Caelli (2001), reduced each transcript to a "story." This procedure was timely but rewarding as 15 stories (ranging from 1 page to 6 pages) were produced from 15 interviews – one per transcript. The advantage of crafting stories is to bring the phenomenon into a clearer focus with a more concise and readable format reducing the need for many pages of interview transcripts to "show" what the researcher is noticing and interpreting whilst remaining true to the data (Crowther et al., 2017). The stories were read again and again, and creative mind mapping became an important activity in making sense of the many parts of the stories. Each story was plotted next to the others in a huge mind-map of pertinent text that had "jumped out" when reading each story. Any text that was similar between the stories was shaded to imply resemblance. Following on from this in a dialectical play between discussions with supervisors, colleagues, family and friends, reviewing the concurrent literature and devising more mind maps on interpretations and thoughts, shared themes began to emerge.

In further dwelling on the analysis, I was struck by how JDM affects the equilibrium of the individual concerned. To a child or young person who is leading a normal, healthy life; to be suddenly knocked off balance by something out of nowhere, which potentially renders them unable to move, was life-changing and was being verbalised in these stories. Seeing this as a metaphor of a rollercoaster helped illustrate this visually, and suddenly all the 15 stories could be plotted together. In keeping with hermeneutic phenomenology, the term *Being* and the dashes between words signify how the *Being-in-the-world* has been distorted from the known, and the journey now is shaped by the phenomena of *Being-on-the-JDM-rollercoaster*.

## Joys, challenges and reflections

Creating the research poems has been a hugely enjoyable and enlightening experience for me. Overall, 16 poems were created, and whilst more than 1 poem was developed from 2 of the transcripts, a further 2 interview transcripts yielded no poems. Whilst this initially caused some personal tensions; I now embrace that this is the beauty of the unbounded nature of hermeneutic phenomenology. The data cannot be manipulated into what it is not. I also recognised how the poems had the potential to invoke distress during dissemination. On reflection, perhaps warning an audience or at least preparing them for what might follow is a good ethical practice. Most importantly, I have been privileged to hear stories from 15 brave and courageous children and young people. My desire is that the findings will not only enhance psychosocial care in clinical practice but also highlight to young people this shared journey that others have taken to lessen some of their uncertainty whilst they ride the JDM rollercoaster.

Hermeneutic phenomenology offers us the opportunity to understand *Being-in-the-world*, especially in times of sickness and ill health. In my study, the metaphor of *Being-on-the-JDM-rollercoaster*, perfectly encapsulates the experiences that the young people were describing. Undertaking phenomenological interviews with children and young people is also not easy, and now I know why there are so few published studies. I would encourage any researcher that would like to conduct hermeneutic phenomenology with children and young people to really take their time to consider how they will get around some of the challenges discussed here. I leave you with a final poem and challenge you to consider what *thrownness* you feel is at the heart of this young person's words:

JDM

Joints, Damage, Muscles
Jolly-well Disappear Musclepain
Jaded, Depressed Moody
Just Disappointing Me
Join Doctors & Mum
Joke, Dumb Mylife
Journey, Diagnosis, Mess ....
.... Anything but Juvenile DermatoMyositis.

## Notes

1. This study has been funded by a National Institute of Health Research (NIHR) fellowship for Health Education England (HEE)/Integrated Clinical Academic (ICA) for non-medical healthcare professionals (Fellowship reference number ICA-CDRF-2016-02-032). PL is also supported by the NIHR Biomedical Research Centre. The views expressed are those of the authors and not necessarily those of the NHS, the NIHR or the Department of Health.
2. This is consistent with the suggestion by Crowther et al. (2017) in their discussion on crafting stories from transcripts in which the authors apply a philosophical perspective to show the incongruence of member checking in phenomenological research.

## References

Ajjawi, R. and Higgs, J. 2007. Using Hermeneutic Phenomenology to Investigate How Experienced Practitioners Learn to Communicate Clinical Reasoning. *The Qualitative Report* 12(4), 612–638.

Apaz, M.T., Saad-Magalhaes, C., Pistorio, A., Ravelli, A., De Oliveira Sato, J., Marcantoni, M.B., Meiorin, S., et al. 2009. Health-Related Quality of Life of Patients with Juvenile Dermatomyositis: Results from the Paediatric Rheumatology International Trials Organisation Multinational Quality of Life Cohort Study. *Arthritis Care and Research* 61(4): 509–517.

Batthish, M. and Feldman, B.M. 2011. Juvenile Dermatomyositis. *Current Rheumatology Reports* 13(3), 216–224.

Bohan, A. and Peter, J.B., 1975a. Polymyositis and Dermatomyositis (Part One). *The New England Journal of Medicine* 292(7), 344–347.

Bohan, A. and Peter, J.B. 1975b. Polymyositis and Dermatomyositis (Part Two). *The New England Journal of Medicine* 292(8), 403–407.

Caelli, K. 2001. Engaging with Phenomenology: Is It More of a Challenge than It Needs to Be? *Qualitative Health Research* 11(2), 273–281.

Carter, B. and Ford, K. 2013. Researching Children's Health Experiences: The Place for Participatory, Child-Centered, Arts-Based Approaches. *Research in Nursing and Health* 36, 95–107.

Clark, A., Flewitt, R., Hammersley, M. and Robb, M. (Editors) 2014. *Understanding Research with Children and Young People*. London: Sage.

Clarke, K. and Iphofen, R., 2006. Issues in Phenomenological Nursing Research: The Combined Use of Pain Diaries and Interviewing. *Nurse Researcher* 13(3), 62–74.

Crowther, S., Ironside, P., Spence, D. and Smythe, L. 2017. Crafting Stories in Hermeneutic Phenomenology Research: A Methodological Device. *Qualitative Health Research* 27(6), 826–835.

Danaher, T. and Briod, M. 2012. Phenomenological Approaches to Research with Children. In *Researching Children's Experience*, edited by Greene, S. and Hogan, D. 284. London: SAGE Publications.

Darmer, P. 2006. Poetry as a Way to Inspire (the Management of) the Research Process. *Management Decision* 44(4), 551–560.

Deakin, C.T., Campanilho-Marques, R., Simou, S., Moraitis, E., Wedderburn, L.R., Pullenayegum, E. and Pilkington, C.A. 2018. Efficacy and Safety of Cyclophosphamide Treatment in Severe Juvenile Dermatomyositis Shown by Marginal Structural Modelling. *Arthritis & Rheumatology* 70(5), 785–793.

Ernste, F.C. and Reed, A.M. 2014. Recent Advances in Juvenile Idiopathic Inflammatory Myopathies. *Current Opinion in Rheumatology* 26(6), 671–678.

Faulkner, S.L. 2009. *Poetry as Method: Reporting Research through Verse*. Walnut Creek, CA: Left Coast Press.

Feldman, B.M., Rider, L.G., Reed, A.M. and Pachman, L.M. 2008. Juvenile Dermatomyositis and Other Idiopathic Inflammatory Myopathies of Childhood. *The Lancet* 371(9631), 2201–2212.

Ferrara, G., Mastrangelo, G., Barone, P., La Torre, F., Martino, S., Pappagallo, G., Ravelli, A., Taddio, A., Zulian, F. and Cimaz, R. 2018. Methotrexate in Juvenile Idiopathic Arthritis: Advice and Recommendations from the MARAJIA Expert Consensus Meeting. *Pediatric Rheumatology* 16(46), 1–14.

Ford, K., Bray, L., Water, T., Dickinson, A., Arnott, J. and Carter, B. 2017. Auto-Driven Photo Elicitation Interviews in Research with Children: Ethical and Practical Considerations. *Comprehensive Child and Adolescent Nursing* 40(2), 1–15.

Gallacher, L.A. and Gallagher, M. 2008. Methodological Immaturity in Childhood Research?: Thinking through "participatory Methods." *Childhood* 15(4), 499–516.

Glesne, C. 1997. That Rare Feeling: Re-Presenting Research through Poetic Transcription. *Qualitative Inquiry* 3(2), 202–221.

Heidegger, M. 2014. *Holderlin's Hymns "Germania" and "The Rhine."* Translated by McNeill, W. and edited by Ireland, J. Bloomington, IN: Indiana University Press.

Hofstager, A. 1988. *Martin Heidegger: The Basic Problems of Phenomenology.* Bloomington, IN: Indiana University Press.

Kim, S., Kahn, P., Robinson, A.B., Lang, B., Shulman, A., Oberle, J., Schikler, E.K. et al. 2017. Childhood Arthritis and Rheumatology Research Alliance Consensus Clinical Treatment Plans for Juvenile Dermatomyositis with Skin Predominant Disease. *Pediatric Rheumatology* 15(1), 110–116.

Kostenius, C. and Öhrling, K. 2009. Being Relaxed and Powerful: Children's Lived Experiences of Coping with Stress. *Children and Society* 23(3), 203–213.

Kountz-Edwards, S., Aoki, C., Gannon, C., Gomez, R., Cordova, M. and Packman, W. 2017. The Family Impact of Caring for a Child with Juvenile Dermatomyositis. *Chronic Illness* 13(4), 262–274.

Laverty, S.M. 2017. Hermeneutic Phenomenology and Phenomenology: A Comparison of Historical and Methodological Considerations. *International Journal of Qualitative Methods* 2(3), 21–35.

Livermore, P. 2014. Juvenile Idiopathic Arthritis: Updated Guide to Administering Methotrexate. *Nursing Children & Young People* 26(1), 26–29.

Livermore, P. and Begum, J. 2021. *Administering Subcutaneous Methotrexate for Inflammatory Arthritis.* 4th edition. London: Royal College of Nursing.

Livermore, P., Eleftheriou, D. and Wedderburn, L.R. 2016. The Lived Experience of Juvenile Idiopathic Arthritis in Young People Receiving Etanercept. *Pediatric Rheumatology* 14(21), 1–6.

Livermore, P., Wedderburn, L.R. and Gibson, F. 2020. You Give Me a Name That I Can't Say, but I Have to Explain What It Is Every Day: The Power of Poetry to Share Stories from Young People with a Rare Disease. *Journal of Poetry Therapy* 33(1), 20–29. doi: 10.1080/08893675.2020.1694210

Lowry, C.A. and Pilkington, C.A. 2009. Juvenile Dermatomyositis: Extramuscular Manifestations and Their Management. *Current Opinion in Rheumatology* 21(6), 575–580.

MacKey, S. 2005. Phenomenological Nursing Research: Methodological Insights Derived from Heidegger's Interpretive Phenomenology. *International Journal of Nursing Studies* 42(2), 179–186.

McConnell-Henry, T., Chapman, Y. and Francis, K. 2009. Husserl and Heidegger: Exploring the Disparity. *International Journal of Nursing Practice* 15(1), 7–15.

McCulliss, D. 2013. Poetic Inquiry and Multidisciplinary Qualitative Research. *Journal of Poetry Therapy* 26(2), 83–114.

Miller, E. 2018. Breaking Research Boundaries: A Poetic Representation of Life in an Aged Care Facility. *Qualitative Research in Psychology* 15(2–3), 381–394.

Mulligan, K., Kassoumeri, L., Etheridge, A., Moncrieffe, H., Wedderburn, L.R. and Newman, S. 2013. Mothers' Reports of the Difficulties That Their Children Experience in Taking Methotrexate for Juvenile Idiopathic Arthritis and How These Impact on Quality of Life. *Pediatric Rheumatology* 11(1), 23.

Öhlen, J. 2003. Evocation of Meaning through Poetic Condensation of Narratives in Empirical Phenomenological Inquiry into Human Suffering. *Qualitative Health Research* 13(4), 557–566.

Page, J. 2018. When Poetry and Phenomenology Collide. *Journal of Aesthetics and Phenomenology* 5(1), 31–51.

Prendergast, M. 2006. Found Poetry as Literature Review Research Poems on Audience and Performance. *Qualitative Inquiry* 12(2), 369–388.

Punch, S. 2002. Research with Children : The Same or Different from Research with Adults? *Childhood* 9(3), 321–341.

Ravelli, A., Trail, L., Ferrari, C., Ruperto, N., Pistorio, A., Pilkington, C., Maillard, S. et al. 2010. Long-Term Outcome and Prognostic Factors of Juvenile Dermatomyositis: A Multinational, Multicenter Study of 490 Patients. *Arthritis Care and Research* 62(1), 63–72.

Shi, Z. 2013. Dilemmas in Using Phenomenology to Investigate Elementary School Children Learning English as a Second Language. *Education* 17(1), 3–13.

Smith, J., Swallow, V. and Coyne, I. 2015. Involving Parents in Managing Their Child's Long-Term Condition – A Concept Synthesis of Family Centered Care and Partnership-in-Care. *Journal of Pediatric Nursing* 30(1), 143–159.

Smythe, E. 2011. "From Beginning to End : How to Do Hermeneutic Interpretive Phenomenology." In *Qualitative Research in Midwifery and Childbirth Phenomenological Approaches*, edited by Thomson, G., Dykes, F. and Downe, S. 35–54. Oxford: Routledge.

Smythe, E.A., Ironside, P.M., Sims, S.L., Swenson, M.M. and Spence, D.G. 2008. Doing Heideggerian Hermeneutic Research: A Discussion Paper. *International Journal of Nursing Studies* 45(9), 1389–1397.

Spence, D.G. 2016. Supervising for Robust Hermeneutic Phenomenology : Reflexive Engagement Within Horizons of Understanding. *Qualitative Health Research* 27(6), 836–842.

Symmons, D.P.M., Sills, J.A. and Davis, S.M. 1995. The Incidence of Juvenile Dermatomyositis: Results from a Nation-Wide Study. *British Journal of Rheumatology* 34(8), 732–736.

Tuohy, D., Cooney, A., Dowling, M., Murphy, K. and Sixsmith, J. 2013. An Overview of Interpretive Phenomenology as a Research Methodology. *Nurse Researcher* 20(6), 17–20.

Walker, W. 2007. Ethical Considerations in Phenomenological Research. *Nurse Researcher* 14(3), 36–45.

Wedderburn, L.R. and Rider, L.G. 2009. Juvenile Dermatomyositis: New Developments in Pathogenesis, Assessment and Treatment. *Best Practice and Research Clinical Rheumatology* 23(5), 665–678.

Wise, B.V. 2002. In Their Own Words: The Lived Experience of Pediatric Liver Transplantation. *Qualitative Health Research* 12(1), 74–90.

# 4 Revealing experiences of sexuality and intimacy in life-limiting illness using Heidegger's phenomenology

Bridget Taylor

## Abstract

My doctoral study sought to understand how people experience sexuality and intimacy when living with a life-limiting illness. The questions I asked and the interpretations I revealed were informed by the philosophical lens of Heideggerian hermeneutics. I interviewed people with terminal cancer or motor neurone disease and, if in a partnered relationship and agreeable, also interviewed their partner. In this chapter, I discuss how Heidegger's philosophy informed the decisions I made in designing and undertaking the study. I reflect on some of the dilemmas I faced and discuss the blind-alleys I went down in attempting to analyse the data. Using interview extracts, I use a paradigm case to demonstrate the constitutive pattern of *Being-towards-death* of the couple. I also describe how Heidegger's views on technology, the concepts of "ready-to-hand," "unready-to-hand," "parts" and "pieces" all helped inform my interpretation of the stories people shared and contributed to their experiences of disconnecting. Finally, I reflect on some of the challenges I faced and how I overcome them when publishing within a field dominated by quantitative research.

## Rationale for undertaking the study

Before embarking on my Ph.D., I worked as a palliative care nurse on a hospice ward and taught sexuality to healthcare professionals in clinical practice and on university courses. Consistent with the literature, I perceived sexuality as a holistic concept that includes how we relate to others but is not dependent on being in a relationship. In my clinical role, I was aware sexuality was rarely discussed; on the occasions when I had broached it with patients, I sometimes uncovered unmet concerns.

At the time, there was a wealth of literature on the impact of cancer and its treatments on sexuality. However, this often focussed on sexual function and sexual satisfaction. There was very little research on the experience of people with terminal cancer or other life-limiting conditions in relation to sexuality. The experiences of partners received scant attention. I wanted to understand how people living with a life-limiting illness experienced sexuality and intimacy to inform palliative care.

DOI: 10.4324/9781003081661-4

## Methodological considerations

Heidegger's philosophy was integral throughout the study's design, informing my research question, approach to data collection, and analysis. His work also provided a lens with which I tried to make sense of people's experiences; to shed light on their life-world. I sought to answer these questions:

- What are the experiences of patients and partners of patients who have life-limiting illnesses in relation to sexuality and intimacy?
- How do people living with a life-limiting illness make sense of these experiences?

## Identifying participants

Because of the wealth of literature on the impact of cancer and its treatment on sexuality, I included people living with motor neurone disease (MND – amyotrophic lateral sclerosis) as this disease process is very different. People with cancer often undergo what they hope might be potentially curative treatment before they receive a terminal diagnosis. In contrast, people with MND are aware their condition is terminal from the point of diagnosis, and their disease results in profound disability. My intention was not to compare these groups but to learn more about the human condition: the shared experience of sexuality while living with a life-limiting illness.

I was mindful of the risk of causing distress by using the term "terminally ill" in any written information, so I opted for "life-limiting illness" as a gentler description. To check whether this terminology was appropriate and the written information clear, I consulted patients with cancer and MND. They endorsed the value of the study and made some useful suggestions for improving the information sheets for potential participants.

## Ethical considerations

I obtained ethics approval[1] and permission from each of the participating organisations. Informed consent, right to withdraw and participants' well-being were paramount considerations. To avoid potential coercion, anyone whose care I was involved in was not invited to participate. To respect confidentiality, I allocated pseudonyms to the transcripts.

## Recruitment

My intention was to interview 20 patients and 20 partners, ten each with MND and life-limiting cancer. I did not require both patients and partners in coupled relationships to participate and included those who were divorced, single or widowed. My aim was to understand the shared experiences of sexuality and intimacy, regardless of relational status; to study Dasein (our awareness of ourselves as human beings) in its *"average everydayness"* (Heidegger 1962, 38).

It is unusual in hermeneutic research to have such a large sample. However, I was mindful that if the findings were to influence healthcare practice, where research quality is often judged by sample size, then larger numbers would be important. I also anticipated a high attrition rate as patients' condition could deteriorate rapidly.

People were eligible to take part if they were over the age of 18, were aware the illness was life-limiting and were able to speak English (to avoid using an interpreter for this sensitive subject). Participants were recruited from clinics, hospice in-patient and day service settings. It proved much harder to recruit partners of patients with cancer as these patients were mostly invited when on a hospice ward or day service and were asked to share information about the study with their partner. This recruitment method proved much less successful than when the partner was present at the time the study was explained; this happened mostly in the MND clinic.

I successfully recruited a range of relationships and a diverse age range (32–82 years). However, apart from one bisexual man and one lesbian woman, the sample was heterosexual. In total, I interviewed 14 patients and 4 partners with life-limiting cancer and 13 patients and 10 partners with MND. Two partners had been bereaved for three months when I interviewed them.

## Gathering the stories in conversation

In my nursing experience, I find that people who describe a very close relationship with their partner often have thoughts, feelings or beliefs they choose not to share as openly with their partner as they might do with someone else. For example, patients and partners tell nursing or medical staff about their worries and fears but may choose not to share them with their partner quite so openly, if at all. Similarly, partners sometimes try to protect their sick partners by hiding their own thoughts and feelings. So that participants could speak freely and not be concerned about their partner's reaction, I chose to interview couples separately (Taylor and de Vocht 2011). I made this clear in the information sheet and reminded people of this when phoning to arrange the first interview.

Given the personal and sensitive nature of sexuality, I anticipated problems with the standard phenomenological question, "tell me about your experiences of ..." I found that most participants were not at ease speaking at length about the subject and required more input from me than might otherwise be expected in hermeneutic research. I asked participants:

- Their reasons for taking part;
- How their/their partner's illness affected them in their day-to-day life;
- Whether this had affected sexuality or intimacy in any way;
- If health care professionals had spoken with them about these matters; and
- If there was anything else, they wanted to share.

The sequencing of these topics was not restrictive but enabled the conversation to move from less sensitive to more sensitive questions and facilitated rapport.

Understanding how illness affected participants in their day-to-day life provided valuable contextual information, as well as examples I could refer back to in relation to sexuality and intimacy. It also enabled participants to talk at length and relax before I moved on to more sensitive questions.

When asked, I did not define sexuality or intimacy; my aim was to enable participants to take the lead on this conversational journey so that issues that were meaningful to them could emerge through the stories they shared. I considered it important to portray openness and acceptance of whatever they said without showing surprise or censor. I encouraged people to speak uninterrupted, though on this sensitive subject, often had to probe for further elaboration. I guided the conversation by returning to points previously mentioned and by asking questions about topics not already described. The interviews, therefore, tended to resemble conversations in that they contained very little pre-determined structure and information was exchanged in both directions. This two-way exchange is consistent with Heidegger's (1962) view that we make sense of our experiences *within* them (as opposed to detached from them). Both I, and the participants, were making sense of experiences "in the world" as they were discussed.

I audio-recorded the interviews, and they were transcribed verbatim. One person with MND communicated using a light-writer, and another used an alphabet board. With their agreement, I repeated their comments aloud during the interview so they could be recorded alongside my own utterances. I was mindful that time was limited for both the patient and their partner, so I decided two interviews would be sufficient to gather useful data without taking up too much of people's time. Because the patients' condition could rapidly change, I arranged the second interview as soon after the first as possible.

Heidegger (1962) recognised that it is impossible to describe without interpretation; human beings live "hermeneutically" as we are constantly interpreting, finding significance and meaning in our worlds. I anticipated that people might not have spoken about many of their experiences before, so the second interview provided opportunities to gather additional information after we had reflected on the first interview. Many participants doubted they had anything to add at the second interview, believing they had already fully described their experiences. However, they elaborated on their previous description, often resulting in richer data. I was also able to pick up on points in more detail without tiring people unnecessarily in the first interview. I did not anticipate that I would learn about conversations that had occurred between partners in relation to the first interview or that a participant would seek permission from someone they were having an extra-marital affair with to describe their shared experiences in the second interview; both provided valuable data.

## Reflexive journaling

Throughout data collection and analysis, I used a reflective journal to record my ideas, impressions and feelings and to question my motives, actions and interpretations. It was important I considered my own position in gathering people's stories and the influence I might have upon the participants and the stories they shared. After all, we co-construct meanings within the world of others.

## Analysis

I adapted Diekelmann's (1992) seven-stage hermeneutic process of analysis to uncover shared meanings. I had to adapt this process because it assumes the researcher will be working within a team, each member independently identifying themes in the data. My Ph.D. supervisors were able to question, challenge and confirm my interpretations, but the responsibility for analysing the data and identifying themes was mine alone.

### The seven-stage hermeneutic process for analysis

Stage 1: I listened to each recorded interview and read through the transcribed text in its entirety to gain a general understanding of each individual's experience. Summarising the interviews was part of this process.

Stage 2: I identified emerging themes within each transcript that reflected meanings in the text.

Stage 3: In meetings with my supervisors, they questioned, affirmed and challenged these interpretations. I returned to re-read the original transcripts and listened again to the interviews when further clarification was needed.

Stage 4: I re-read all of the transcripts to identify common themes, and began to explore these themes through writing, using excerpts from the transcripts, exemplars and "paradigm cases" (an account offered by one participant that is a particularly strong instance of a theme present in multiple transcripts).

Stage 5: I identified a "constitutive pattern" (the highest level of hermeneutic understanding). This pattern describes the relationship among the themes across all the transcripts.

Stage 6: I compared the transcripts, looking for similar or contradictory interpretations of the emerging themes and constitutive patterns. I discussed these themes and the pattern in a variety of forums (including clinicians, academics, patients, relatives) to challenge and further develop my interpretations.

Stage 7: I returned to the philosophical and theoretical literature to further refine my interpretations within a broader context.

In a dialectical play, moving backwards and forwards between the interviews, I checked to see whether other narratives supported or refuted any emerging themes. This iterative process illustrates the hermeneutic circle of interpretation whereby understanding the "whole" requires reference to the individual "parts" and understanding each "part" requires reference to the "whole" (Figure 4.1) with reflection integral throughout.

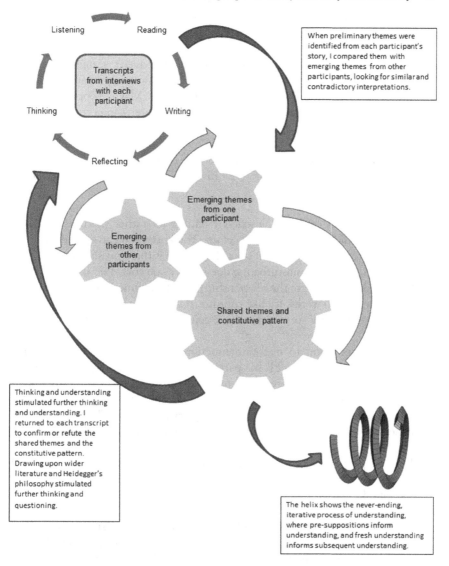

Listening    Reading

Transcripts
from interviews
with each
participant

Thinking    Writing

When preliminary themes were
identified from each participant's
story, I compared them with
emerging themes from other
participants, looking for similar and
contradictory interpretations.

Reflecting

Emerging themes
from one
participant

Emerging
themes from
other
participants

Shared themes and
constitutive pattern

Thinking and understanding
stimulated further thinking
and understanding. I
returned to each transcript
to confirm or refute the
shared themes and the
constitutive pattern.
Drawing upon wider
literature and Heidegger's
philosophy stimulated
further thinking and
questioning.

The helix shows the never-ending,
iterative process of understanding,
where pre-suppositions inform
understanding, and fresh understanding
informs subsequent understanding.

*Figure 4.1* The Iterative Process of Hermeneutic Understanding

Through reflection, it occurred to me that none of the participants had mentioned masturbation or using sexual aids unless I directly invited them to. On the occasions when I asked about these means of sexual expression, many participants were very willing to share their experiences without further prompting. My initial interpretation was that participants' silence reflected a higher level of sensitivity for sexual practices that carried a taboo; I believed I had given them permission to speak the unspeakable. However, I was also mindful that what emerges in good phenomenological interviews is what is meaningful to participants. From my journal:

> Is it really just a matter of sensitivity? People haven't seemed any more uncomfortable telling me about their experiences of masturbation or using sexual aids than when they shared anything else. Maybe people don't volunteer these experiences because, for them, they aren't important means of expressing sexuality or intimacy.

This became clearer when I returned to the narratives. For example, Sean described the benefits of masturbation for his confidence but recognised it did not provide what he needed:

> It's the intimacy and the closeness I hanker for rather than just the sex, because I could go anywhere and get sex. You know, you can go and pay for it down the road, you could … it's not that side of it that's missing, but the intimacy and you know, masturbating doesn't give you that. But also, after what happened at the start of the relationship [erectile dysfunction], it just gives me confidence it still works. It's like running. If you go out running, you know, if you stop running for six months, you're going to struggle when you start again.

Sean used masturbation to maintain function; it provided reassurance of his ability to have intercourse with his partner, but it was not a substitute for the intimacy he craved. When I returned to the data, I began to more fully understand the experience of "masturbation as a poor substitute for connecting" (Taylor 2012). As Jim explained: "it's a poor second, a very poor second."

Further understanding began to dawn some months later, as my journal shows:

> It seems people understand sexuality and intimacy to be embodied, sexual experiences. I now realise this began to show itself in the reasons people gave for *not* taking part in the study:
>
> > I don't feel my input would be of any benefit to your study. Any sexual or intimate contact stopped long before my husband's diagnosis. I would like to have helped if circumstances were different. (*Tina*)

Participants who were single, divorced and widowed told me their life-limiting illness rendered them no longer eligible for sexuality or intimacy:

> How does a bloke, why would he want to get into a relationship with a single woman who has got a life-limiting illness? You're not going to be a really good catch, are you? (*Kim*)

I should not have been surprised at this as being-with is a mode of Dasein's being; we are always in relation with others, and our everyday way of being-in-the-world is one of engagement (Heidegger, 1962). In the context of sexuality and intimacy, these participants reminded me we are inescapably social beings, always in relation with others, always being-with.

I did, however, go down several blind alleys in my analytical attempts. I initially tried using NVIVO software to code the transcripts. Not knowing what was important, I coded almost everything. Although partly beneficial, as it helped draw out the impact of equipment on intimacy and sexual expression (Taylor 2011), I was concerned this resulted in descriptive rather than interpretive analysis. I found the software reductionist as it drew me to focus on detail. I was in danger of over-looking the whole experience by focussing on snippets, so abandoned it at an early stage.

I understood that summarising the narratives could be a useful way to understand people's experiences. My attempts at these written summaries were extremely time-consuming and largely unproductive. This was partly due to my inexperience but also because the narratives were so rich that I did not want to lose anything. While some of the summaries were helpful, many were barely shorter than the interviews themselves. I found it particularly helpful to hear myself summarise the narratives when talking with my supervisors and fellow students. Through sharing participants' stories and trying to do justice to their experiences, they began to become a little clearer for me.

My next attempt involved gathering all the extracts from the interviews that related to one topic. Heidegger (1962) used the example of a hammer to explain how entities are understood in relation to each other. A hammer is understood in relation to its purpose of banging in a nail, and the nail is understood in its purpose of connecting two pieces of wood in order to construct a building. The building is understood in terms of the purpose it serves in keeping animals dry or in providing a home. Meaningfulness is therefore established in terms of its function and purpose: "in-order-to" and "towards-which" (Heidegger 1962). In the context of my study, this is exemplified in terms of a bed:

> A bed is a bed because of the meaning it holds for us; we might understand it as a place to sleep, or as a place to be intimate, or indeed as a place to die.
>
> (Taylor and de Vocht 2011, 1579)

We turn towards a bed because of the function it holds for us. This may be in-order-to have sex, in-order-to sleep or in-order-to rest when unwell. It is the in-order-to and for-which that determine meaning (Heidegger 1962).

I sought to understand what sexual intercourse meant for people by gathering together the descriptions relating to sexual intercourse (see Table 4.1). Considering function and purpose, I was able to group these into themes according to the meanings sexual intercourse held for people.

As my journal extract shows, this raised further questions:

> It's gratifying both men and women seem to cherish an emotional connection through sex. It's sad that, for some, this is now missing. But what about the people who did not talk about sex? I can't ignore their narratives. Is there something shared in their experiences alongside people who did speak about it? What about those who were not in a relationship?

*Table 4.1* Some emerging themes relating to sexual intercourse

| Examples from the narratives | Emerging theme |
|---|---|
| Jim: *It was like breathing … natural and beautiful and a joy.* | Sex as part of life |
| Maureen: *I haven't, as yet [since the operation], felt comfortable with having sex, I haven't felt … it's more of a chore rather than a pleasure.* | Sex to be endured |
| Tom: *Our sexual relationship has not been fantastic, probably for about 14, 15 years, I mean it's something that's been very much sort of once a month, maybe twice a month, you're my husband, it's my duty … She denies me what really a couple should be doing for one another. I think it's a huge part of a relationship. I don't see why I should be denied our sexual relationship.* | Sex as a right/ duty/obligation |
| Tom: *It certainly takes your mind off other things that are going on.* | Sex as therapy |
| Sharon: *He says it doesn't worry him, but I know that all men, I mean he's still a fairly young man so I'm sure it must, he must still get the urge to have sex even though he doesn't force himself on me at all, but I just feel I need to let him have sex … I can't say that I'm enjoying it, but I do it for Tony.* | Sex as a gift for the other |
| Bert: *Like all married couples, we occasionally disagree about things you know, and we don't have that avenue [sex] of making up any longer. So, you have to be a bit more careful in our diplomacy, shall we say.* | Sex as repair |
| Tom: *Making love is about two people, it's not about one.* | Sex as mutuality |
| Nick: *It is part of keeping bonding together, isn't it? It's always something that has been important to us, so if it's taken away from you then it would be; the partnership would be obviously changing.* | Sex as bonding |
| Michelle: *The feeling that having sex brought me was just a constant reminder that I was going to lose that person soon … obviously I didn't want to upset him by saying that, because it was like reminding him, you know, you're dying.* | Sex bringing the future into the present |

I decided to set aside my written words (in the form of codes, summaries and preliminary themes) and, instead, to dwell in the data. I listened to the interviews and re-read the transcripts multiple times, pondering what people had shared. I was surprised how useful it was to re-play the interviews and hear people share their stories again and again. The nuances in their delivery were not adequately represented in the written transcripts. It was through familiarity that I was more able to hear what they were telling me. When I tried too hard to make sense of the narratives, it was unproductive. Insights often came when I allowed the data the freedom to speak: participants' stories would come to me when I was walking or swimming. I was more able to understand their experiences when I wasn't focussed on trying to categorise them; analysis could not be rushed.

I was advised that some journals required the use of a software package in analysing data, so did make a further attempt at using NVIVO once clearer themes had emerged. At that point, I knew the narratives so well this was somewhat superfluous.

Diekelmann (1992) advocated returning to participants to confirm interpretations. However, hermeneutic phenomenologists hold differing views about this process of "member checking." Some see this as a way of improving trustworthiness; others contend it is only the researcher who is exposed to the myriad horizons of understandings shared between participants, the literature, and their own background of understanding. Apart from checking my emerging understanding from what participants had shared in the first interview at the second interview, I considered member checking problematic (with similar views expressed elsewhere, for example, by Polly in Chapter 3). I anticipated that many patients would not be alive or well enough when I was at this point in the process. I was also aware many of the partners would have been bereaved (and possibly in a new relationship). It was likely, therefore, that participants' perspectives on sexuality and intimacy would have altered since the data were collected; this would have resulted in them interpreting their prior words from a new position (Taylor and de Vocht 2011).

## Insights gained from Heidegger's philosophy

Heidegger's philosophy was integral to the analysis. I found his ideas challenging and grappled to understand some of his concepts, while others resonated more easily and provided valuable insights. As shown above, his discussion of function and purpose ("in-order-to" and "towards-which") prompted me to consider the meanings sexual intercourse held for people. Several Heideggerian concepts were integral to analysis in my thesis (Taylor 2012); some extracts are included here.

When initially reading Heidegger's (1977) work on technology, which draws on hydroelectric power as an example, I saw no connection to sexuality and intimacy and almost disregarded it. In my struggle to understand his texts, I drew on my own examples to try and understand his ideas more easily; reciprocally, his work provided a lens through which I viewed the data.

Heidegger (1977) viewed technology as more than a means-to-an-end, he saw it as a way of revealing (also discussed in the context of education by Margot in Chapter 8 and in the context of birth stories by Lesley Kay in Chapter 5). When we focus solely on what technology can do (its promise), we are blind to the threat it poses; we therefore need to understand both the enabling and disabling effects of technology.

Unprompted, participants described their experiences of different technologies including the hospital bed and speech assistive devices. Some participants spoke about the technological changes to their body as a result of reconstructive surgery, while others described their experiences of using the medication, Sildenafil.

Through Heidegger's work, I came to understand Sildenafil as a medicinal "tool" that chemically engineers an erection; it is prescribed by doctors to fix the faulty machine (the penis). However, as Clive explained, Sildenafil merely enabled the penis to be "ready for use":

We occasionally get it together [have intercourse] but it's a bit of an effort ... I got some Sildenafil and we've used that once or twice with varying success (laughs). It works in terms of, you know, creating the erection, yes, but if other parts of the ol' system aren't equally excited, shall we say, then it won't necessarily result in the outcome that you hope it will.

Sildenafil served a purpose in enabling Clive to have intercourse with his wife, but when he was not adequately aroused himself, he did not achieve orgasm. Sildenafil can also create an expectation of sexual intercourse that, as Katy explained, is not always willingly reciprocated:

> I could be *so* tired and then he'd come up and he'd just want to have sex. And I'm not somebody who would just, you know, say, 'No, I'm sorry [Jake], I'm not having it' because I don't like to reject somebody. But then he'd go, 'that was a waste of a tablet', and then I'd feel really *bad* and, oh okay … there were times when I just didn't want to. He would come to bed late and I'd be half asleep and I'd have to get up early in the morning for the boys and he'd want it, and he'd have taken a tablet without telling me. So, he'd still have it.

Katy described a lack of shared decision-making: her partner did not consult her before taking Sildenafil and expected her to have intercourse, whether she wanted to or not, to avoid wasting a tablet.

According to Heidegger (1977), the issue with technology is the objectification of Being; under its reign, everything comes to exist as ready for order. In other words, modern technology looks to manipulate nature, to impose on it; to undermine its ontological and structural integrity in multitudinous ways such that we can demand more of it. Heidegger (1977) believed we need to open up the possibility of relying on technologies while not becoming enslaved to them. I found his work helpful in understanding the order imposed upon the body through technology. Sildenafil worked by calling Jake's body to action, and therefore, both his and his partner's bodies were positioned as "standing reserve" (an orderly resource required to be available and respond in a specific way for a particular purpose). By positioning bodies as standing reserve, their natural resources are revealed and therefore controlled, ordered, and exploited:

> Through revealing the body and its processes in particular ways, other facets and processes become concealed.
>
> (Zitzelsberger 2004, 247)

When Jake took Sildenafil and presented his body ready for intercourse, the lack of intimacy within their relationship was concealed when Katy acquiesced. Through sharing her experience, their way of *Being-in-the-world* with each other and the lack of intimacy and equality in their relationship were revealed.

The narratives revealed that Sildenafil did not facilitate connecting; the human body became objectified and phallocentric notions of sex were reinforced at the expense of intimacy and connecting. The essence of their sexual relationship (connecting through mutuality) was lost when the erect penis became a "piece" rather than a "part":

> The piece [*das Stück*] is something other than the part [*der Teil*]. The part shares itself with parts in a whole. It takes part in the whole, belongs to it. The piece on the contrary is separated and indeed, as the piece, is even isolated from the other pieces. It never shares itself with these in a whole.
>
> (Heidegger 2012, 34)

Sildenafil is the agent by which a "part" is rendered a "piece." When taking Sildenafil, the erect penis becomes ready and available for intercourse. However, the chemically induced erection is not "part" of the experience of connecting; it is merely a "piece" whose integrity is missing. For these participants, using Sildenafil was experienced as disconnecting.

Having explored participants' narratives about Sildenafil, I became aware that others also spoke about the disruptions they had experienced to their body's integrity. Angela told me she had insisted on a breast implant when she had her mastectomy 15 months previously:

Angela:  It's no longer a breast; it's a prosthesis, really, which just happens to be inside my skin … I think it's affected my confidence. I knew he found my breasts attractive, so it was something I was quite happy to show off and be in a position where he could appreciate what they looked like. And now on occasions, although he doesn't say anything and he doesn't seem to find them, it, unattractive, it just goes through my mind if we're being intimate, this must look ridiculous … it's not the same visual impact at all that it used to be and I'm very conscious of that.

Bridget:  Is that because of the nipple missing or is it more than that?

Angela:  It's more than that. It's because the nipple is missing but also because they just don't move in the same way. It's a breast form, you know, it's not a replacement breast, it's a breast form … in some ways with my clothes on it's an improvement … I actually think in terms of proportion, now I look better with my clothes on … but certainly with my clothes off I don't like how I look … if it's affecting anything it's the intimacy with me and my husband … I need more reassurance now … I'll get undressed and I'll turn around and I'll look at him and I'll say … 'don't you think that it looks really ridiculous?' … He doesn't really enter the discussion; he always just says 'you're fine. You're lovely to me' and that's it.

Heidegger (1962) referred to our taken-for-granted way of *Being-in-the-world* as "ready-to-hand" (Lesley Dibley also offers further consideration of this

Heideggerian notion in Chapter 6). When we become aware of what is broken or missing, this heightens our awareness of what we do have and results in us missing even more what is not within reach. What we do have is seen in a new light, deficient in the shadow of what it could be if what is unavailable were to be present. Therefore, it is only when something fails in its purpose (at times of breakdown) that it becomes conspicuous and the taken-for-granted meaning is exposed.

Angela's breast had been surgically replaced "in-order-to" resemble the breast that had been removed and "for the sake of" appearing normal. Under technology's pervasive rule, everything becomes replaceable. However, Angela's breast was not replaceable. Surgery had rendered the "breast form" no longer fit for purpose. Although she felt it was an improvement to her appearance when clothed, the breast form was conspicuous and obtrusive during sex with her husband, Angela's attention was drawn to it, and it was no longer "ready-to-hand":

> It revealed itself as a something just present-at-hand [a breast form] and no more.
>
> (Heidegger 1962, 103)

Angela's loss of her breast was not necessarily about role or function. Her breast was symbolic of the taken-for-granted sexual relationship she and her husband once shared. The playfulness in their relationship was gone because her breast form was obtrusive during these intimate moments:

> [In the past] If I didn't have my nightie on, I would sit up and I knew that he found it quite attractive to be able to look up at my breasts. But that's a thing I never do now.

Angela's breasts were an important component of her sexual relationship with her husband. The absence of one breast, and its replacement with a breast form, was experienced as disconnecting within her sexual relationship as she felt "ridiculous" in her disfigured body. Her husband's behaviour also changed in response to this prosthesis:

> He doesn't tend to touch the breast form … he tends to only touch the left breast. It makes me feel if I ever have to have that removed, what then? Then there'd be nothing left and how would he feel about that? And how would I feel about that? … When we go to sleep, I lie on my left side and he always puts his arm round me and his arm always comes to rest there. And I'm very conscious of the fact there is only one … I'm conscious of thinking thank goodness at the moment that still feels the same.

When her husband touched her healthy breast, the presence of his touch reminded Angela of her missing breast. She was also aware of the fragility of this touch, and the fragility of her body, as there might come a day when that breast also had to be removed. Her husband's reassurance that she was "fine" was ineffective because she was reminded of all she had lost. Their sexual relationship had lost its spontaneity and playfulness, and even sleeping side by side brought the future into the present, reminding her of what might yet come.

For Angela, the artificial breast was only a piece of her; it did not belong to her body in the way a nose belongs to, and is part of, the face and completes the whole. Unlike cosmetically enhanced breasts that are a matter of choice, surgery for breast cancer disrupts the body's integrity; the breast form that was created to replace Angela's diseased breast was not a "part" of her. Its relationality determined whether it was a piece or a part – its relationality in the context of her body and in the context of her sexual relationship with her husband.

## Identifying a paradigm case and constitutive pattern

The experiences described above brought me closer to an understanding of disconnecting within the coupled relationship. Throughout the analysis, I checked and re-checked that I had not excluded any of the narratives. One participant's interviews troubled me greatly. Tom had shared detailed descriptions of his extra-marital sexual relationship and his earlier loss of virginity. I doubted the relevance of these stories as they occurred before his diagnosis. I was struck that he didn't appear embarrassed or regretful; he seemed almost gleeful, maybe even lascivious. I wondered if he was trying to establish some sort of sexual bond with me and felt very uncomfortable. I had been concerned about my safety.

It is not always possible at the time to know if an interview is productive, but I knew my analysis would be influenced by my emotional responses. Through journaling, I reflected on my conflicting feelings and tried to understand Tom's motives for sharing these stories. I became more aware of my prejudices and the influence of these pre-suppositions on my interpretations:

> I feel antipathy towards Tom as a sexual being and wonder if his wife has felt the same? I wonder if his descriptions of what I think of as irrelevant experiences will prove to be a turning point in my analysis?

It was only after I processed my feelings about this interview that I was able to understand the significance of his descriptions. It was through empathy and trying to understand the meaning these other sexual experiences held for him and their relevance when he knew he was dying that enabled me to see for the first time the connection he missed within his marriage and found in his extra-marital relationship. This journal entry shows the progress I made in my journey towards understanding:

> In describing his relationship as "a ninety-five per cent marriage" Tom felt deprived; cheated of one of life's great pleasures. He described his extra-marital

sexual encounters as fulfilling because, with her, he achieved the intimacy that he craved. Unlike his wife, his sexual partner reciprocated his sexual advances and achieved sexual satisfaction. For Tom, her responsiveness was as important as his own sexual pleasure.

As I rightly surmised, his interviews were a turning point in my thinking; Tom's narratives turned out to be an important paradigm case. This is an account provided by one participant that is a particularly strong instance of a theme that is present across multiple narratives. Tom described "sexuality and intimacy as disconnecting," which revealed itself as:

- Disconnecting as a legacy from the past (pre-existing sexual difficulties impeding connecting);
- Disconnecting as rejection;
- Disconnecting as lack of reciprocity;
- Disconnecting as rights and duties.

(Taylor 2012, 86)

For Tom, sexuality and intimacy were also experienced as "re-connecting in the shadow of impending death" during what he described as an "intense period of sex" with his wife in the week immediately after his diagnosis (Taylor 2012). The constitutive pattern of "Being-towards-death-of-the-couple" reveals itself in the following extracts. By applying stage 5 of the seven-stage approach, you can discern how the following extracts describe the relationship among the themes across all the transcripts. Diekelmann (1992) contends that this is the highest level of hermeneutic understanding.

### The constitutive pattern of "being-towards-death-of-the-couple" reveals itself

When you're sleeping in a double bed and the other person's got her back to you and doesn't want to know and you're sort of pushed across, there is a form of, there is a feeling of rejection ... you just go through that little period of time before sleep takes over where everything goes round in your mind and then you think back 20 years, 25 years when things were really brilliant and wishing it to happen again ... It [sex]'s something I need and it's something that I can't have and it's something I can't do anything about ... I didn't feel that before, I mean before the diagnosis, if we had situations like that, well it was just, you know, things haven't changed, maybe they will next time ... I feel that time is running out, whereas before I felt things were good once and things can be good again, and there's plenty of time to get that right ... and that's not going to happen, because who knows how quickly this is going to take my life away from me. (*Tom*)

If I think about it [the future] too much I get very sad because we don't have a future anymore. (*Julie*)

He'll come and give me a little peck on the cheek and he tells me he loves me, and I know he loves me dearly but ... the cuddling and the kissing's gone ... The close relationship you get just to kiss and cuddle and, in the end it's ... We're slowly dying a sort of death really. (*Kathleen*)

## Lessons learned from publishing the findings

I considered it very important to publish my findings in journals accessed by healthcare professionals caring for people with MND and terminal cancer. After all, my intention in undertaking this research had been to inform clinical practice. The review process helped me clarify concepts that might otherwise puzzle or confuse a reader; things that I implicitly understood but had not adequately explained for others. Looking back, I realise that if I had been more confident, I might have been more able to successfully argue my corner and avoid making some of the compromises I did. One of the biggest constraints was the limited permitted word count. Reviewers were often unfamiliar with the methodology and requested further detail. This meant compromises at the expense of discussing my own position as a gatherer of people's stories. I wonder now whether I could have included extracts from my journal in a figure, unconstrained by the word allowance.

In my experience, quantitative ideals were often evident in reviewers' comments. For example, some challenged my use of the first person, suggesting I wrote in the passive voice. In one journal, I was able to successfully argue that referring to myself as "the researcher" when reflecting on my role in gathering people's stories was inconsistent with the methodology. I conceded in the rest of the article and used the passive voice, though have wondered since whether I could have resisted this compromise. Another example is when I was asked to demonstrate that interpretations were validated by multiple-rater agreement with "two researchers coding separately, and then comparing results and discussing any discrepancies." This had not been possible as my supervisors had different expectations. Instead, I tested the emerging themes at the second interview and presented my interpretations to a variety of audiences. Many people have since told me they have "heard" their own experiences in the data. I successfully argued that the echoes of my interpretations in the experiences of others affirmed my emerging understandings and provided a "hallmark of trustworthiness" (Smythe et al. 2008, 1396), which is consistent with this methodology.

Another reviewer asked me to justify why I did not use a structured interview schedule, suggesting this limited the generalisability of the findings. I successfully explained that the findings from hermeneutic phenomenology are not intended to be generalisable and that the unstructured interview format is consistent with this methodology in order that experiences that were meaningful to participants could freely emerge. When challenged, I have successfully justified why I did not return the findings to participants for confirmation for both ethical and methodological reasons. I had concerns about compromising confidentiality and causing distress as patients' health was likely to have declined in the intervening time.

Also, if participants had read the transcripts after the interview, they would have been reading them in a different context to when their words were originally spoken, and their reading would have produced new interpretations of meaning.

I have learned through the publishing process how important it is to clarify the expressions of rigour that guided the study and that they are consistent with the methodology.[2] It has been helpful to explain Heidegger's (1962) stance that understanding is always "on the way"; there is always the potential for new findings to emerge from data. There is no such thing as one correct interpretation; it is just *an* interpretation. Findings are merely interpretations that present "a calling, an invitation to others to come and look and think" (Smythe et al. 2008, 1393).

## Final reflections

I have asked myself many times whether I needed to have interviewed such a large sample. Although this enhanced the credibility of my findings for clinical practice, where quantitative ideals and sample size are important, interviewing 41 participants, 34 of whom I interviewed twice, resulted in an enormous amount of data. If I had interviewed a much smaller sample, as is more conventional in phenomenological research, I might have been able to overcome some of the difficulties I experienced summarising the narratives.

While each person's story helped illuminate the experience of sexuality and intimacy when living with a life-limiting illness, some described experiences not evident in other narratives:

> Situations like this uncover long wounds that have grown up, but they also can be very healing in some aspects. I wouldn't say it's all negative. (*Frances*)

A smaller sample might not have revealed the experience of re-connecting these few participants described. By comparing and contrasting the narratives and searching for shared experiences, any differences I encountered caused me to question and challenge my emerging understanding. Including people who were not in a coupled relationship was valuable in revealing sexuality and intimacy as embodied, relational experiences.

If I had chosen to limit the study to one illness, it is likely my findings would have been different. By choosing to include two different illnesses and interviewing both patients and partners, I have revealed something of the human condition. There is no such thing as one correct interpretation; the prism of people's experience has many facets. The ones described here are not all there is to this aspect of these participants' relationships; they are what called to me as they shared their stories at the time in which they did.

Heidegger's philosophy constituted part of my fore-structure of understanding. I am not familiar with all his work and am by no means an expert. What I have attempted to show here is how some of his ideas helped on my journey towards understanding.

# Conclusion

In this chapter, I have attempted to demonstrate the thinking and doing of this study and to show how the decisions I made were underpinned by the philosophical lens of Heideggerian hermeneutics as I moved towards an understanding of what it means to be human and experience sexuality and intimacy when living with a life-limiting illness.

The experience of being human is dynamic and complex. A life-limiting diagnosis disrupts the life course for the person who is dying and brings with it an irreversible end to human bonds. The prism of people's experience has many facets. The ones described here are not all there is to this aspect of these participants' relationships; they are what called to me as they shared their stories at the time in which they did. In the end, the reader must decide on the trustworthiness of my phenomenological interpretations.

The understanding I have gained from undertaking this work brings with it a sense of seeing anew. However, the cyclical process of interpretation and understanding is never-ending, for the understanding of what it is to be human is always "on the way" (Heidegger 1962). In our never-ending circle of interpretation, the end is to go back to where we started:

> We shall not cease from exploration
> And the end of all our exploring
> Will be to arrive where we started
> And to know the place for the first time.
> (Eliot 2001, 43)

## Notes

1. Ethics approval: National Health Service (NHS, UK) ethics committee approval (study number 08/H0603/3).
2. I adopted the framework developed specifically for hermeneutic phenomenology by de Witt and Ploeg (2006).

## References

de Witt, L., & Ploeg, J. (2006). Critical appraisal of rigour in interpretive phenomenological research. Journal of Advanced Nursing, 55(2), 215–229.

Diekelmann, N. (1992). Learning-as-testing: A Heideggerian hermeneutical analysis of the lived experiences of students and teachers in nursing. Advances in Nursing Science, 14(3), 72–83.

Eliot, T.S. (2001). Little Gidding. In T.S. Eliot (Ed.), Four Quartets (pp. 33–43). London: Faber and Faber.

Heidegger, M. (1962). Being and Time. Oxford: Blackwell Publishing.

Heidegger, M. (1977). The Question Concerning Technology and Other Essays. New York: Harper Collins.

Heidegger, M. (2012). Bremen and Freiburg lectures: Insight into That Which Is and Basic Principles of Thinking. Translated by A.J. Mitchell. Bloomington, IN: Indiana University Press.

Smythe, E., Ironside, P., Sims, S., Swenson, M., & Spence, D. (2008). Doing Heideggerian hermeneutic research: A discussion paper. International Journal of Nursing Studies, 45(9), 1389–1397.

Taylor, B. (2011). The impact of assistive equipment on intimacy and sexual expression. British Journal of Occupational Therapy, 74(9), 435–442.

Taylor, B. (2012). Couples living in twilight: A Heideggerian hermeneutic study of sexuality and intimacy in life-limiting illness. Unpublished doctoral dissertation, Oxford Brookes University, Oxford. Available: https://radar.brookes.ac.uk/radar/file/862e3752-0cd2-a088-3a90-880de1b7a46c/1/taylor2012couples.pdf

Taylor, B. (2014). Experiences of sexuality and intimacy in terminal illness: A phenomenological study. Palliative Medicine, 28(5), 438–447.

Taylor, B. (2017). Using Heideggerian hermeneutic phenomenology to understand sexuality and intimacy in life-limiting illness. In SAGE Research Methods Cases. London: SAGE Publications Ltd. https://dx.doi.org/10.4135/9781526408013

Taylor, B., & de Vocht, H. (2011). Interviewing separately or as couples? Considerations of authenticity of method. Qualitative Health Research, 21(11), 1576–1587.

Zitzelsberger, H. (2004). Concerning technology: Thinking with Heidegger. Nursing Philosophy, 5(3), 242–250.

# 5 'Distracted by, and immersed in the talk of others'

## Expectations and experiences of childbirth in the framework of the "They"

*Lesley Kay*

## Abstract

In this chapter, the underpinning thinking, design, conduct and findings of a hermeneutic phenomenological study, underpinned by Heideggerian philosophy, are used as a vehicle to demonstrate a means of researching, interpreting and understanding complex phenomena. Specific focus on the philosophical notions of the "They," "authenticity" and "idle talk" are presented as ways of illuminating meaning. As a woman, a mother, a midwife, a researcher and a lecturer I carried out a study which sought to determine how other women's birth stories construct and reconstruct the meaning of birth for childbearing women. I start the chapter by revealing the significance of the subject area, moving on to explain how I developed the research design. I outline my interpretive process relating to some of the joys and challenges of adopting that process. I illustrate the process by sharing "Stephanie's story" and, in doing so, hope to guide the reader contemplating a similar journey. I conclude the chapter by reflecting on how the work has influenced me and my subsequent research and practice.

## Significance of the birth story

Childbirth is a momentous event in a woman's life and one that can assume enormous psychological importance (Callister, 2004), and the birth story as "*a feminine, woman-to-woman legacy*" is understood as a crucial source of knowledge about childbirth for mothers (Savage, 2001; Humenick, 2006; Nichols, 1996). Articulating the birth experience into a story gives it structure; once the experience has a structure, there is potential for meaning to be determined and emotional responses considered (Farley and Widmann, 2001).

My interest in the birth story started with the idea that for millennia stories have been used as a means of understanding and learning, and an awareness that the story, and the teller, undoubtedly influence us as we try to 'make sense' of a situation (Frank, 2010). I was of the mind that birth stories must surely have a positive or negative influence on listeners, and those stories, and the messages they transmit, must therefore have the potential to steer women either towards or away from medical and/or midwifery-led models of care.

Certainly, I came to the study with a certain amount of 'fore-understanding' about childbirth and about the experience of women engaging with birth stories

DOI: 10.4324/9781003081661-5

whilst they are pregnant (Smythe and Spence, 2012, 16) (also discussed by Liz and Deb in Chapter 2). At the outset of the process, I was interviewed by two of my supervisors about my presuppositions. This excerpt from the interpretation of my pre-understandings interview in 2012 reveals a starting point:

> Throughout my personal interview I assert that women are 'dictated to', 'fed' and 'subliminally told' about birth purporting my belief that childbirth in the UK is conducted and organised in an autocratic manner. I talk about 'the doctor', 'the hospital system', the concept of safety and medicine expressing the belief that birth is 'less and less about women', the suggestion being that the pervasive understanding of birth in this society is founded on a socially constructed, biologically determined and medically managed ideology.

I recognised that I was grounded in a particular conception of both birth and the birth story:

> I am grounded in my conception based on my experience of already being in the world of birth. I am a woman who has heard stories of birth, a mother who has birthed, a midwife who has attended countless births and a lecturer who has read and taught around the subject of birth. I am skilled at existing in this world and am therefore caught in the swirl of existence I am hoping to understand.

From my practice as a community midwife, my own experience of birth as 'normal', and my belief that most women, if cared for appropriately, can birth physiologically, my conception of birth is most definitely in the naturalistic "camp" as opposed to that of the medical. Being grounded in a conception is not unusual. Heidegger reminds us that no interpretation of an object can ever be free of preconceptions because, without some preliminary orientation, it is impossible to grasp the object at all. Heidegger argues that *"every inquiry is seeking"* and that *"every seeking gets guided before-hand by what is sought"* (2012, 24).

### Finding resonance with a research design

Having noted that hermeneutic phenomenology had been successfully utilised in several midwifery studies (Hunter, 2008; Thomson, 2007; McAra-Couper, 2007), I started to explore the feasibility of using the approach in my study. The process of realising hermeneutic phenomenology described by Smythe et al. as *"a journey of 'thinking' in which researchers are caught up in a cycle of reading-writing-dialogue"* (Smythe et al., 2008, 1389), appealed to me much more than an overly prescribed methodology.

I saw a resonance between the practice of midwifery, which embraces a holistic philosophy in which midwives are encouraged to "be with woman," caring for women within the context of their lives and according to their individual needs, and the methodology which enables the researcher to "be with the data." Others have also noted how hermeneutic phenomenology is resonant with mid-wifery ways of knowing (Miles et al., 2013). Birth does not happen in a vac-uum separated from the world but is lived and breathed by the birthing woman and her midwife. Similarly, thinking and writing for the hermeneutic researcher appeared all encompassing; grounded in an understanding of the social, emo-tional, cultural and spiritual experiences of the participants and the researcher (Smythe et al., 2008).

Initially nervous about using the approach because of its strong philosoph-ical foundation and the fact that there was not a fully developed and system-atic method to employ, I was excited by the apparent "freedom" the approach promised and the opportunity for reflective thinking. By utilising a hermeneutic phenomenological framework, I hoped to understand women from "inside" their subjective experience and to find insights that applied more generally to empha-sise what we may have in common as human beings.

At the beginning of my journey, I attended the "Institute for Heideggerian Hermeneutical Methodologies" in the United States. Within a community of other beginners, I learnt about the approach, writing an "I" poem (inspired by the work of Gilligan, 1982) to demonstrate my first tentative understandings of using hermeneutic phenomenology as a research methodology:

*I have a voice*

I see, but do I see?
I am a fish, but I do not see the water
I cannot hope to understand you because I know too much
I have my own 'gaze', but I also have a sense of 'it'
I am not the expert
I inhabit my world
I am engaged openness
I see through my past in the present and in my future
I am a living, ontological being
I am skilled at existing
I am ready to hand
I understand and yet I do not
I will come to understand
I am always already in the world
I am caught in the swirl of existence that I am trying to understand
I need to listen to what is said
I need to listen to what is not said
I am always already in the world of birth
I am a co-participant
I must ask the right questions
I will understand what I am thinking when I see what I write
I will have many conversational partners
I will get a glimpse

I will pull out what catches my 'gaze'
I will hammer out my idea
I am exposed, vulnerable, open, and raw
I am excited by possibility
I feel it!
I get it!
I finally trust it
I am honoured to be part of it
I anticipate a 'luscious mess'
I must read into this
I must read out of this
I will reveal the concealed
I feel empowered
I will find meaning right in front of me
I will make a case and I will invite you in
I am open to possibilities and to mysteries
I will make an interpretive leap but will not have a firm footing
I am approaching an abyss
I am looking for what lies near
I want to share
I want to have a voice
I want to tell a story.

## The study

My overarching research question was: "*How does engaging with stories of birth help pregnant women to understand what their experience of birth may be?*" To enable me to understand the experience of women engaging with birth stories whilst pregnant with their first child, I purposively selected and interviewed 20 U.K. participants. Findings from an initial sample of ten pregnant women indicated that virtual media was a primary source of birth stories. Conversations with these women led to questions about whether the information gleaned from media and virtual birth story mediums creates meaningful knowledge about birth for women. The second phase evolved from this thinking. In phase two, interviews with an older cohort of women (who were pregnant in the 1970s–1980s) were undertaken to determine whether women from a different era were more able to translate knowledge into meaning. This was based on the belief that, for this generation of women, stories were mediated by personal contact and not through virtual technologies as in the previous generation of women.

## Interpretive process

Without a clear set of procedures, it follows that the hermeneutic phenomenological process is enacted differently by every individual researcher; rather than being a series of steps to be followed, the researcher is always in the "midst," going backwards and forwards between the literature, the participants, the "stories" and evolving insights. Smythe et al. (2008, 1391) describe this space as *"the leeway,"* the space *"between structure and freedom."* In this space, the research *"is the writing"* and in the thinking, there are no *"subheadings"* by which to classify or arrange our thoughts (Smythe, 2008, 228). My interpretive process was informed by the processes of Van Manen (1984) and Smythe (2003, 2011). Unpacking the meanings hidden in the women's stories was iterative and prompted by a series of questions, adapted from Smythe's work (see Table 5.1), which I used to stimulate thinking and writing.

*Table 5.1*  Writing and rewriting

| Writing and rewriting – working with the data | |
|---|---|
| **Clarifying pre-understandings – at the outset and throughout** | What is my understanding? How will my understanding effect my interpretation? |
| **What is my response to this transcript?** | Get a sense of the bits you respond to |
| | Recognise the phrases that leap out and grab you |
| **What things jump out?** | Find what matters |
| **"Dwelling" with the data** | Be attentive to the research question |
| | Find the pieces that have something important to say |
| | Gather the meaning together |
| **Find resonance in the literature** | Think about the context of what you are interpreting; this will help you to see meaning and significance |
| | Read the literature but also read fiction to help you understand and conceptualise ideas and notions |
| **Helping the data to speak** | Find the meaning threaded through |
| **1. Writing a summary** | Write a summary of what the participant said so that the reader can share your focus |
| **2. Move to interpretation** | Think about the meaning that lies behind the saying |
| | Craft a story from the transcript |
| **3. Invite other voices in** | Think about what the literature says about the phenomena |
| | Are there any exemplars in art, poetry or prose? |
| | Write in response to your growing understandings |
| | Rewrite the story |
| **4. Bring in philosophical and phenomenological notions** | Add a philosophical lens and make an "interpretive leap" |
| | Elucidate possible meaning by relating it to Heideggerian notions |
| | Write in response to your growing understandings |
| | Rewrite the story |
| **Pulling it all together** | Let the themes emerge |
| | Select the best stories to illustrate a theme |
| | Write, drawing on the stories, interpretations, voices from the literature and Heideggerian notions |
| | Form an argument that expresses the meaning of your phenomenon |
| | Write clearly and simply to allow the meaning to "leap off the page" |

Source: Adapted from Smythe (2003, 2011).

## Unpicking the interpretive process: Stephanie's story

With the above steps suggested by Liz Smythe in mind, this section illustrates my interpretive process by sharing how I responded to and worked with Stephanie's interview transcript. I started by considering my response to her transcript, thinking about the things that jumped out, whilst remaining attentive to the research question and the text that seemed to have something important to say about the phenomenon. Different types of story segments from Stephanie's transcript that jumped out are illustrated in Table 5.2.

## Dwelling with the data, gathering the meaning together and writing a summary

After immersing myself in the data, I started to gather the meaning together, writing the following:

> Stephanie talks about her understandings of birth and where those understandings have come from. She recalls being a child and remembers women in her family having babies; seeing them with 'ashy' faces, getting up 'gingerly' and having 'hushed conversations in the corner' all gave her an impression of how bad birth was. As she got older Stephanie recalls stories about how 'rough it was', how 'sore' women felt afterwards and how 'long' it took to recover from birth. The stories from Stephanie's family were all about situations being completely outside of their control; about it all being a 'rush' and 'major panics'. Stephanie tells me that the stories you hear make it feel like it's all out of your hands and that you go in, and basically, you're in there for hours, and everything kind of happens at once and the nurses, or whoever, take over.

The stories Stephanie has heard as an adult have mostly been "horror stories"; the oh my god it's so painful, it's so awful, you just kind of want to forget about it kind of stories. Stephanie tells me that positive stories rarely get told and that it would be worth saying if things are not "too bad" rather than always perpetuating the "horror" stories which circulate so readily. Stephanie compares telling such stories to writing reviews on something like "Amazon," saying that although some people put up good reviews, most of the people who put a review on do so because it is negative.

Stephanie says that you do not appreciate how much information about birth gets "filtered in" through the years; for instance, the expectation that childbirth hurts, but don't worry, you'll forget, and you'll come out the other side of it. Stephanie tells me that her perception had been that "you get on a bed" and that your birth on the bed, something which she thinks probably came from things that people had told her and photographs she had seen of women sitting in bed cradling their newborn babies.

Before attending National Childbirth Trust (NCT) classes and aqua natal classes, Stephanie had no appreciation that she would be able to make choices

Table 5.2 Things that jumped out from Stephanie's story

| | | | | | | |
|---|---|---|---|---|---|---|
| **Stories shared** | Stories I've heard were all the "oh my god it's so painful, it's so awful, you just kind of want to forget about it" kind of stories | The stories you hear, make it feel like it's all out of your hands – you go in, basically you're in there for hours, and everything kind of happens at once and the nurses, or whoever, take over | All the stories are about how rough it was, how sore and how long it took to recover | They're the only stories you seem to get – you don't get anyone who says "it's brilliant, calm and relaxed." You just get these horror stories | The people who go into it are the ones who have the horrific stories … its almost kind of cathartic … they have to keep telling it and they have to tell you | And it's all you know, "well, we managed to get through it but, you know it was 30 odd hours of absolute hell and you know, I don't quite know how I got through it and the end and everything else"… and you think "oh god that's what I've got to look forward to" |
| **Family stories** | Stories from my family were about things being completely out of their hands – it was all a rush and all major panics and upset | People in my family said that they might decide it would be easier to do a C-section | When I was a child and people in my family had babies …. I saw them kind of getting up gingerly, and it was all hushed conversations in the corner which gave an impression of how bad it was | After my nephew was born, I saw my sister and she was just kind of ashy | My mum was a midwife, and she has very set ideas – I grew up with the view that you need to try and do everything for yourself because it's not good to have intervention | |

(Continued)

Table 5.2 Things that jumped out from Stephanie's story (Continued)

| | | | | | | |
|---|---|---|---|---|---|---|
| **Friends stories** | Friends have told me you just get through it and you know it's all worth it | People who have positive stories don't want to kind of go into it | One friend of mine had quite a long labour but she was … all the way through everything, whatever happened, she was always amazingly happy about everything | Everything was kind of real gushy … and I was like "yeah, I'm sure it wasn't because it was just … everything was perfect and wonderful?" | | |
| **Information about childbirth** | The more I read the more conflicting it gets, the more confused I get and the more I just really don't want to know because I just think well, I don't know now – I've got to the point where I don't want to read anymore because I've reached saturation | I've reached overload and I don't know what's going on in my head – I think there's too much out there at the moment | You can buy something from Amazon, you've got reviews. Some people put up good reviews but most of the people who put a review on is because it's negative | You don't think about how much of it gets filtered in and through the person's experience | But it's also the fact that the consensus is it hurts, but don't worry, you'll forget, and you'll come out the other side | It's probably worth saying if things aren't too bad rather than letting everyone just get on with this … yeah it's absolutely terrifying, it's awful, but don't worry, you forget – that's what you get told, that's the message |

(Continued)

Table 5.2 Things that jumped out from Stephanie's story  (Continued)

| Beliefs about childbirth | I was anticipating that, because of the problems with my pelvis, a lot of it would be out of my hands | There's also a sense of naivety about it – you fall pregnant, it's all fine and then you have the baby | As I say I didn't think it'd be so much kind of choice that it'd be very much, well, you do what we say, you breathe when we say and then, kind of we see what happens and decisions get made | I thought there wouldn't be a lot of choice because it didn't sound like there was with the births that I'd known most about | Even knowing what I did I still thought you get on a bed at the end and someone kind of coming out through your legs and up in the air and everything – I think you get that idea from what people say and photos you see straight afterwards | I've been into hospital many times for operations and normally you go in, you get told where to go, they do everything for you now – so when you're pregnant you think surely they'll do the same thing because you're in a hospital – professionals will probably tell you – we want you like this |
|---|---|---|---|---|---|---|
| Preparation classes | NCT and aqua yoga classes have changed my views about birth | It is all about relaxation – If you relax you can control the pain a lot more | The classes have taught me that I can do a lot to make it what I want – I had no idea before that | But the classes have made me question that – it's even been suggested that I could have almost "a kind of semi-enjoyable delivery" – mind you everybody still says it's not! | I thought it would be that it would just happen and I wouldn't get a choice but I now know they can't tell you, it's your decision and you've got to keep it in your control | |

and decisions and take control over what happens during her baby's birth. Rather she thought that it would be more like you do what we say, you breathe when we say, and then, kind of we see what happens and decisions get made. Having been into hospital many times, Stephanie assumed that her experience would be similar; you go in, you get changed, you get told where to go, and they do everything for you.

Stephanie describes attending the NCT classes and aqua natal classes as having changed her views. Stephanie has learnt the value of relaxation and the benefits of water for weightlessness and movement and now feels reassured that she can do a lot to make the birth what she wants. She recognises that she can be involved in planning the birth and in considering choices and making decisions arising during her labour and birth. Stephanie feels a sense of control over the process, which she did not have before.

## Helping the data to speak – moving to interpretation

Stephanie's first understandings of birth were based on what she had witnessed as a child, heard people talk about as she grew up, what she imagined from pictures and television programmes, and what she had deduced from stories she had been told.

Her perception was also based on her experiences of hospital admissions for surgery; where you attend, get changed into a hospital gown, get onto a bed and staff do everything for you. She imagined that during birth surely, they'll do the same thing because you are in a hospital. This is a valid deduction to make; Stephanie is used to handing over responsibility for herself and her body when she enters a hospital. She anticipates that the professionals know the correct course of action to take and believes that they will always act in her best interests. Nothing in her experience to date has led her to question this.

Stephanie describes, with some surprise, her belief that knowledge and/or information has "filtered through" over the years almost without her realising it. Until our conversation, Stephanie had not really considered how she knew what she did about childbirth; her understandings and expectations were just there in the background. As she describes it, "knowledge" and "understanding" of birthing is seemingly all around and is passively absorbed into human consciousness by a process akin to osmosis.

Stephanie's experience of stories is primarily of the "horror" type of story. Despite wanting to hear more positive stories, Stephanie appears sceptical when she recalls a positive story as it does not fit with her preunderstandings of birth. Again, this is unsurprising if stories such as this are completely at odds with her perceived understandings of birth as something painful, long, arduous and which necessitates you to "get over it" and "forget it."

Attending classes has changed Stephanie's "views about birth"; Stephanie has learnt the value of relaxation and the benefits of water for weightlessness and movement and now feels reassured that she can do a lot to make the birth what she wants. Stephanie's experience is a positive one; she recognises that she can be involved in planning the birth and in considering choices and making decisions arising during her labour and birth. Stephanie feels a sense of control over the process, which she did not have before.

Stephanie has been given a lot of information and told that she can be instrumental in her own birth; she wants to believe this and to experience a birth which is "almost enjoyable" rather than having an experience which is akin to those of members of her family. She remains slightly sceptical, however, as everything she believed prior to the classes is at odds with what she now "knows." She has obviously discussed what she has "learnt" with others and still has a concern about the role of the professional in her care; despite being told that choices and decisions will be in her control, she is worried that this will not be the case. Why should she put faith in what she has heard in the classes if everything she thought she knew and everybody else's opinion is at odds with this?

## Helping the data to speak – finding resonance with other sources

Next, I thought about what the literature had to say about the phenomena by reading around the subject matter. I added a philosophical lens to make an "interpretive leap" relating what I was writing to the Heideggerian philosophy underpinning the study, specifically Dasein and Being-in-the-world. I utilised a mapping document (Table 5.3) to help me identify the notions which spoke to the emerging meanings. Through mapping emerging meanings, it became evident that the philosophical notions of authenticity, The They and idle talk were key to illuminating the phenomenon of the study. These notions are in quote marks in Table 5.3 to signal the principal notions explored in this chapter.

Stephanie's pre-understandings are rooted in her experience of "being-in-the-world" of birth; she experiences aspects of this world in relation to other people in that world. In Stephanie's case, these people are members of her family and her close friends. In her pregnancy, Stephanie finds herself in a world that appears to operate in a certain way and where certain things have already shown up as important. Heidegger describes this as "*thrownness*," explaining that Dasein is "*thrown*" into its "*there*" (Heidegger, 2012, 173). As "thrownness" Dasein finds itself already in a certain moral and material, historically conditioned environment (also discussed by Polly, Chapter 3 and Lesley Dibley, Chapter 6). Using this lens, women are "thrown" into the world of birth; once in this world, women are faced with an array of possibilities or choices which are somehow limited. Women, therefore, choose possibilities of action that are conditioned by their enculturation into the practices of their specific childbearing community.

Stephanie, for example, has been born into a family in 21st century Britain, a family, whose experience of birth, is that of it being out of your hands and of people taking over. Thrown as she is into this world, Stephanie attunes herself, creating her existence in terms of what she sees as possible. Stephanie, as "*everyday being-with-one-another*" is dependent on others, and the "They" inconspicuously dominate the way to be (Wrathall, 2005, 686).

*Table 5.3* Mapping emerging meanings with Heideggerian notions

| Emerging meanings | Philosophical notions |
| --- | --- |
| • Protecting or neglecting<br>• Shrouded in mystery or blissful ignorance<br>• Conspiracy of silence | • In our everyday lives we do what "one" does according to the norms laid out by the "anyone" of which we are a member – authenticity – conformity – the "They"<br>• Lostness in the "They"<br>• "Disburdened" by the "They" |
| • Horror stories/making people feel bad<br>• Too perfect and wonderful<br>• Offering platitudes<br>• Avoiding the gory bits | • "Thrownness" – women "thrown" into the world of birth, choose possibilities of action that are conditioned by their enculturation into the practices of their specific childbearing community<br>• Authenticity – conscience – guilt<br>• Care – as Dasein's act of expressing anything about itself to itself – our interaction with things in the world – dimensions of "authentic" and "inauthentic" existence<br>• "Leaping in" and dominating – where one cares for the other by simply taking up that other's burden and doing it for them, for example, by not providing information leading to women feeling out of control when birth is not as expected/medical professionals "taking care" of women |
| • Media portrayal<br>• The "modern birth story"<br>• Going the opposite way | • Idle talk – the way of speaking within the framework of the "They" – a way of speaking which controls and levels out all interpretations of the world – accepting what is claimed, simply because it is said, and passing it on, further disseminating the claim |
| • Knowledge and information filtering through | • Authenticity<br>• Leaping ahead' and liberating – "where the other is helped to take up their own burden by giving them the means to bear that burden on their own" (such as through providing information/birth planning/raising awareness of difficulties that could present) |

## The They, inauthentic and idle talk

Heidegger's concept of the "They" alludes to the community into which we find ourselves thrown. It is a *"primordial publicness"* that serves as a shared basis for *"everyday understandings"* (Bessant, 2011). In our everyday lives, we do what "one" does according to the norms laid out by the "anyone" of which we are a member. Griffiths suggests that the "They" presents each Dasein with *"specific, ready-made, acceptable, moulds, opinions and attitudes that are deemed correct, to ensure the well-being of the 'they' as a totality"* (Griffiths, 2009, 113).

Our competence in coping with the world, therefore, is of a tacit attunement to cultural practices. Heidegger describes our everyday *"being-in-the-world"* as our *"dealings in"* the world arguing that we are so absorbed in the world that we do not consciously interpret or attribute meaning to anything around us (2012, 95). Rather we take for granted and do not question the "normal" situatedness of our being:

We take pleasure as they take pleasure; we read, see, and judge about literature and art as they see and judge; likewise, we shrink back from the 'great mass' as they shrink back ... Everyone is the other, and no one is himself. The 'they', which supplies the answer to the 'who' of everyday Dasein, is the 'nobody' to whom every Dasein has already surrendered itself in being-among-the-other.

(Heidegger, 2012, 165–166)

Stephanie's world of birth is an experience of being in a world populated by doctors and technology; all in place to safely "manage" her well-being and her birth. In Heidegger's view, the human way of being is incomprehensible in isolation from a grasp of the world in which it "is." Dasein exists in an environment in which it is *"tempted, seduced, soothed or estranged"* by the world around it (Harman, 2007, 30). The childbearing woman can never just "be" within the world of birth without already being a part of it and potentially being "spoiled" by it.

Being "spoiled" by the modern technological world is something which concerned Heidegger as he believed that technology held more danger than potential and had the capacity to obscure the meaningful presence of things; he spoke of the modern world as a world where things show up as having the potential to be ordered according to the norms of control and efficiency of that world (Heidegger, 1954) (also discussed by Bridget, Chapter 4, Margot, Chapter 8). In this world, people share a way of "being" with all other "things" and are therefore prized in terms of their ability to function as another "resource."

In this world, the "They" disburdens Dasein in its everydayness because it never faces the responsibility of its own choice. According to Heidegger, the "immediacy and perplexity" of Dasein's existence is lost and covered over by allowing the "They" to remove its responsibility for being. He characterises this mode of being as inauthentic or fallen, arguing that we live inauthentically when we function in our everyday existence as part of "the-They,"

... in the practical public environment, in utilising public means of transport and in making use of information services such as the newspaper, every other is like the next. One's own Dasein dissolves completely into the kind of being of 'the others.'

(Heidegger, 2012)

In the everydayness of living our lives, we just get on with and do the things that we need or want to do. Dasein loses sight of itself when it "falls into" and is immersed in the world, neglecting itself as an autonomous individual and interpreting itself purely based on its situation and preoccupations (Inwood, 2000).

Stephanie's attunement to birth is reinforced by the "received knowledge" (Belenky et al., 1986) she encounters in the form of the stories she hears, which add emphasis to her understanding of birth as being "*so painful ... so awful, you just kind of want to forget about it.*" This is because much as they are "thrown" into a particular world of birth, women also "fall" into the dialogue and speech of that world, with what is talked about becoming normative, widely accepted, and gaining authority (Griffiths, 2009). This means that what is shared and heard about birth is not innocuous, as beliefs which are groundless and without any real content become prevalent influencing behaviour and understandings.

Heidegger uses the term "Gerede" ("idle talk") to describe the way of speaking within the framework of the "they" (Heidegger, 2012). Idle talk is a way of speaking which controls and levels out all interpretations of the world, it is *the form of intelligibility manifest in everyday linguistic communication - average intelligibility*" (Mulhall, 2013). We accept what is claimed simply because it is said, and we pass it on, further disseminating the claim (Heidegger, 2012).

In a world where the public way of understanding birth (the "painful, awful" horror stories as described by Stephanie) is disseminated so widely, women may find themselves "*taken in a peculiar direction and …. absorbed in the immediate, in fashions, in babble*" (Heidegger, 2002). Being caught up in the "hype" around birth could mean that women understand "what is said-in-the-talk" but that what the talk is about is "understood only approximately and superficially" (Heidegger, 2012). The inference being that women in today's "world of birth" may be approaching childbirth with an average understanding of the claims about birth as opposed to a genuine understanding of birth itself.

Stephanie would like to hear more positive stories of birth, as opposed to the "horror" stories she describes. Despite wanting to hear more positive stories, Stephanie appears dubious when she recalls a positive story. This is unsurprising as stories such as this are completely at odds with her perceived understanding of birth as something painful, long, arduous and which necessitates you to "get over it" and "forget it."

After hearing countless "horror" stories positive stories are not accepted as "real life." More than that, because of human beings "everydayness" and "absorption" in the world, what is extraordinary (the "horror" of birth described in a story) is made ordinary through familiarity; the appearance of "horror" in a story is accommodated and then made invisible by that accommodation, whilst other interpretations are effectively "closed off" (Heidegger, 2012). In effect, the idle talk that is shared about birth appears to close off possibilities for women to view or understand birth in any other way; their experience of stories does not speak to the genuine nature of birth or its possibility for being something other than a "horror" to be endured and put to one side as they embark on mothering.

After attending classes, Stephanie recognises that she can be involved in planning the birth and in considering choices and making decisions arising during her labour and birth. Stephanie feels a sense of control over the process, which she did not have before. Her perspective has changed, and she sees new possibilities of interacting with others; Heidegger describes this type of interaction as "*leaping ahead*" and "*liberating*," as something we do for the "*other*" in our being with (Heidegger, 2012, 159). By attending classes and working with other members of the group and the facilitator, Stephanie is able to confront what she thought she knew about birth and learn how to exert control over her experience. This means that she sees the potential to experience a birth which is "almost enjoyable" rather than having an experience which is akin to those of her family members.

Despite her newfound understandings, Stephanie remains slightly sceptical as everything she believed prior to the classes is at odds with what she now "knows." She has obviously discussed what she has "learnt" with others and still has a concern about the role of the professional in her care; despite being told that choices and decisions will be in her control, she tells me that "everybody still says it's not!" Why should she put faith in what she has heard in the classes if everything she thought she knew and everybody else's opinion is at odds with this? Stephanie struggles with the idea that her experience can indeed be different.

Heidegger believes that people have a natural inclination to conform because, ultimately, they want to become accepted in their community. Their other option, "mineness," recognising their own possibilities, which are not shared by others, carries the risk of them feeling alone and possibly ostracized. Perhaps Stephanie does not really believe in her ability to experience a different kind of birth, or maybe she has not got the courage to claim the possibility of being instrumental in her own birth?

## Moving from interpretation to the phenomenon

Stephanie's story was one of 20 stories within which the phenomenon of birth stories was buried. The phenomenon revealed itself tentatively at first; hidden as it was within the experiences of each individual woman. As I started to consider the data as a whole and invited other voices into the phenomenological conversation, commonalities started to appear allowing the phenomenon to move out of the shadows into what Heidegger describes as the "clearing" (Heidegger, 2012). In my writing, I articulated the meanings that emerged from my thinking and reading; these meanings formed the threads of the thesis.

The threads of the thesis spoke of stories as problematic for the women in the study, of a prevalence of "horror" stories and of a scepticism around positive birth stories. Further, they spoke of the notion of birth as something "which must take its course" and where women must concentrate their energies on "coming out the other side." Taken as a whole, the threads of the thesis revealed that the information gleaned from birth stories did not, in fact, create meaningful knowledge and understanding about birth for these pregnant women. Instead of helping women to prepare for birth, the stories shared made women fearful of birthing, persuading them that birth was a "drama" to be navigated and forgotten and an endeavour for which they lacked the necessary knowledge and skills. Seeking "sanctuary" from the "drama" of birth, many of the women appeared to persuade themselves they would be more "secure" within the system of birth where accountability rested with the experts.

In conclusion, I argue that the idle talk around the experience of birth potentially causes pregnant women harm, disempowering them and denying them possibilities for an alternative birth. The potency of idle talk in the narration of birth stories, therefore, holds significance for us all in the "The They" of our existence.

## Reflecting on the journey

My hermeneutic phenomenological journey was at times arduous, taxing, exhilarating, creative, "freeing," frightening, overwhelming, but ultimately enriching. I learnt about my strengths: strong organisational skills, the capacity to work independently and to sustain motivation and momentum, and the ability to work to deadlines, and my weaknesses: letting the best be the enemy of the good and the art of procrastination. At the end of the process, I remained invigorated by the ideas which motivated me at the outset and by the notion that women intuitively know how to birth.

## Conclusion

My experience of applying this methodology has, I believe, helped me to a better question, listen, think and write about any phenomenon I am studying. As a researcher, I am always absolutely and concretely at the heart of any study that I undertake. In designing, conducting, interpreting, and writing up, I rely on my own experiences of womanhood, pregnancy, birthing, midwifery and storytelling to help me engage with the study, the participants and the conversation. Throughout the process, I kept a reflexive journal, and in my finished thesis, added excerpts from my reflexive writing, providing an audit trail of my engagement and impact on the research, signposting the reader to my research journey.

I end by offering a final "I" poem as a gift of knowing to those who follow in my footsteps and embark on a hermeneutic study of their own. The poem tells of my journey, of what I found and what inspires me as I continue my practice as an educator and a researcher. I encourage researchers who undertake a hermeneutic study to be open to possibilities, to question, to listen, to read widely, engaging with the arts, poetry and prose, to write and rewrite and to be courageous enough to take an interpretive leap.

> *Everydayness, absorption and the 'idle talk' of birth*
>
> I wanted to tell a story
> I was interested in meaning and in birth
> I thought that storying was significant
> I knew everyone had a story to tell
> I was excited about understanding and engaging with stories of birth
> I wanted to live the experience
> I wanted to listen and to learn
> I took part in the phenomenological conversation
> I started to see how it could be being-in-the-world-of-birth
> I acknowledged many story mediums
> I called them the modern birth story
> I was inspired by storying power
> I knew a story could be a spark
> I heard about the horror
> I heard about the drama

I heard nothing of joy or of physiological birth
I watched as women tried to understand
I felt their need to know
I noticed everyone wanted to share, partake and be part of the story
I recognised the fascination
I saw the energy and risk of sensationalism
I remembered the feeling of fear
I remembered worrying about death
I remembered the questions without answers
I knew about the uncertainty
I knew about the pain
I observed how stories could devastate
I appreciated how stories could transform
I wanted women to value the journey
I saw them race to the end
I thought we have taught them to question
I thought we have said we offer choice
I thought we have told them what and where
I thought but we have not told them how
I wanted them to know their power
I wanted them to believe in their strength
I wanted them to be primal and I wanted them to be proud
I knew women felt there was a right way
I saw them struggle to be good
I watched them try to be compliant, to try and follow the rules
I heard them doubt their own bodies, their own knowledge and strength
I listened as they tried to imagine
I watched as they sought, and they sought
I saw how they turned to the experts
I knew they did it to feel certain and be safe
I was saddened by the stories
I heard the same formula again and again and again
I recognised the same narrative script, the long and short of it
I saw women absorbed in the immediate, in fashions and in babble
I knew they were caught up in hype
I saw the extraordinary made ordinary
I saw other interpretations closed off
I watched them float in the shelter of gossip
I watched them bolstered by Heidegger's 'idle talk'
I saw birth was a paradox, a mystery waiting to be solved
I saw that the storying needed to be positive, capable, loud, and proud
I saw women needed nurturing and ultimately to be heard
I finally understood women need to believe in birth.[1]

# Note

1. Ethics was obtained and approved by the University of Central Lancashire (UCLan) BuSH (Built, Sport and Health) in 2012 (phase 1) and 2014 (phase 2).

## References

Annells, M. 1996. Hermeneutic phenomenology: philosophical perspectives and current use in nursing research. *Journal of Advanced Nursing* 23: 705–713.

Belenky, M.F., B.M. Clinchy, N.R. Goldberger and J.M. Tarule. 1986. *Women's Ways of Knowing: The Development of Self, Voice, and Mind* (Vol. 15). New York: Basic Books.

Bessant, K. 2011. Authenticity, community, and modernity. *Journal for the Theory of Social Behaviour* 41, no. 1: 2–32.

Callister, L. 2004. Making meaning: women's birth narratives. *JOGNN: Journal of Obstetric, Gynecologic and Neonatal Nursing* 33, no. 4: 508–518.

Farley C. and Widmann, S. 2001. The value of birth stories. *International Journal of Childbirth Education* 16: 322–325.

Frank, A.W. 2010. *Letting Stories Breathe: A Socio-narratology*. Chicago: University of Chicago Press.

Gilligan, C. 1982. *In a Different Voice*. Cambridge, MA: Harvard University Press.

Griffiths, D. 2009. Daring to disturb the universe: Heidegger's authenticity and the love song of J. Alfred Prufrock. *Literator* 30, no. 2: 107–126.

Harman, G. 2007. *Heidegger Explained: From Phenomenon to Thing*. Chicago: Open Court.

Heidegger, M. 1954. The question concerning technology. *Technology and Values: Essential Readings* 99–113.

Heidegger, M. 2002. The principle of identity. In *Identity and Difference*. Translated by J. Stambaugh. Chicago: University of Chicago Press.

Heidegger, M. 2012. *Being and Time*. Oxford: Basil Blackwell.

Humenick, S.S. 2006. The life-changing significance of normal birth. *Journal of Perinatal Education* 15, no. 4: 1–3.

Hunter, L. 2008. A hermeneutic phenomenological analysis of midwives' ways of knowing during childbirth. *Midwifery* 24, no. 4: 405–415.

Inwood, M. 2000. *Heidegger: A Very Short Introduction*. Oxford: Oxford University Press.

Kay, L. 2016. Engaging with the 'modern birth story' in pregnancy: A hermeneutic phenomenological study of women's experiences across two generations. Doctoral dissertation, University of Central Lancashire.

Kay, L., S. Downe, G. Thomson, and K. Finlayson. 2017. Engaging with birth stories in pregnancy: a hermeneutic phenomenological study of women's experiences across two generations. *BMC Pregnancy and Childbirth* 17: 283.

McAra-Couper, J. 2007. What is shaping the practice of health professionals and the understanding of the public in relation to increasing intervention in childbirth? Ph.D. diss., Auckland University of Technology.

Miles, M., Y. Chapman, K. Francis, and B. Taylor. 2013. Exploring Heideggerian hermeneutic phenomenology: A perfect fit for midwifery research. *Women and Birth* 26(4): 273–276.

Mulhall, S. 2013. *The Routledge Guidebook to Heidegger's Being and Time*. New York: Routledge.

Nichols, F.H. 1996. The meaning of the childbirth experience. *The Journal of Perinatal Education* 5, no. 4: 71–77.

Palmer, R. 1969. *Hermeneutics Interpretation Theory in Scleiermacher, Dilthey, Heidegger and Gadamer*. Evanston: Northwestern University Press.

Parsons, K. 2010. Exploring how Heideggerian philosophy underpins phenomenological research. *Nurse Researcher* 17, no. 4: 60–69.

Savage, J. 2001. Birth stories: a way of knowing in childbirth education. *Journal of Perinatal Education* 10, no. 2: 3–7.

Smythe, E. and D. Spence. 2012. Re-viewing literature in hermeneutic research. *International Journal of Qualitative Methods* 11 (1):12–25.

Smythe, E. 2011. From beginning to end: how to do hermeneutic interpretive phenomenology. In *Qualitative Research in Midwifery and Childbirth: Phenomenological Approaches*, edited by G. Thomson, F. Dykes and S. Downe. London: Routledge.

Smythe, E. 2003. *Getting Going: What Is the Meaning of the Experience of Driving Home from Work?* Unpublished manuscript.

Smythe, E., et al. 2008. Doing Heideggerian hermeneutic research: a discussion paper. *International Journal of Nursing Studies* 45: 1389–1397.

Thomson, G. 2007. A hero's tale of childbirth: An interpretive phenomenological study of traumatic and positive childbirth. Ph.D. diss., University of Central Lancashire.

Van Manen, M. 1984. Practicing phenomenological writing. *UALibraries Site Administrator Test Journal* 2, no. 1: 36–69.

Wrathall, M. 2005. *How to Read Heidegger*. New York: W. W. Norton and Company.

Wrathall, M. 2013. *The Cambridge Companion to Heidegger's Being and Time*. New York: Cambridge University Press.

# 6 Seeking Heidegger in research data

## Thinking about connections between philosophy and findings

*Lesley Dibley*

### Abstract

In this chapter, I present a study exploring the meaning of the experience of kinship stigma in people with inflammatory bowel disease (IBD). We used individual unstructured hermeneutic interviews to collect data from 18 UK-dwelling participants. The phenomenon of kinship stigma (feeling stigmatised by close or intimate family members) was first identified in my PhD and challenged Goffman's assertion that "the Wise" (those with a special or privileged relationship with the marked person) would be supportive. A key tenet of hermeneutic phenomenology is the use of one's own – and others' – existing knowledge and experience within the study. We research the experiences that interest us *because* of who we are, not *despite* who we are. This invites a certain way that acknowledges the significance of where we are situated within a study yet also guides us to manage the pre-understanding/prejudice we bring with us. Through reflection (looking back on a past event) and reflexivity (an active self-awareness of one's own judgements, beliefs and perceptions during an event), we demonstrate the credibility and trustworthiness of our work.

## Introduction

In hermeneutic phenomenology, we also draw on others' knowledge and experience – typically through reference to other published works – to illuminate meaning for the reader, but may overlook the opportunity to draw on Heidegger's philosophy to help "show forth" the meanings within our data and offer these to others for their consideration. In this chapter, I explain how I came to do the kinship stigma study and how, in a secondary analysis of the data, the following three Heideggerian notions helped reveal another interpretation of the meaning:

- **Pre-understanding**: the knowledge which exists before we fully understand it, which influences understanding and beliefs, and which we bring with us and draw on to make sense of new situations.
- **Thrownness**: our past is always before us: our historicity gives us a starting point such that we have somewhere or something that we come from and are already determined in where we go to.
- **Ready-at-hand/unready-at-hand**: the taken-for-granted availability of "things" which go unnoticed, until these become unavailable.

DOI: 10.4324/9781003081661-6

I begin by reflecting on some aspects of my life story and my prior engagement with phenomenology and stigma theory that led me to the study before demonstrating how bringing Heideggerian notions with us into analysis adds philosophical depth to what "shows forth."

## My pre-understandings

I started my professional life as a Registered General Nurse caring for adults before specialising as a Registered Sick Children's Nurse in the mid-1980s, moving into nurse education in the mid-1990s, and eventually finding my current home as an academic researcher in 2008. Throughout my nursing career, I developed an abiding interest in the everyday world of chronically sick individuals. I was also attracted, undoubtedly due to my identity as a gay woman, to the notion of "Other." Phenomenologically, the "Other" refers to recognising another as different from oneself and incorporating one's understanding of this difference into one's own sense of self – by recognising that we are a different person from the other, we come to understand who we are ourselves (Hegel 1770–1831). Psychologically and sociologically, "Othering" refers to identifying those not belonging to the (majority) in-group and using the differences to reinforce positions of preference, power and superiority (Canales, 2000; Johnson *et al.*, 2004). Othering is closely linked to prejudice, discrimination and stigmatising attitudes (Young-Bruehl, 1996) and has, historically, been used in many contexts such as male dominance (McCann & Kun, 2003), HIV/AIDS (Petros *et al.*, 2006) and those with non-heterosexual identities (Carpenter, 2018). Since my first undergraduate dabble in research in the early 1990s, I had developed an interest in Heidegger's interpretive phenomenology. Via an MPhil phenomenological project on lesbian women's experiences of healthcare (Dibley, 2009) and extensive reading, I recognised that this philosophy reflected my own way of being in the world – all of which created a momentum such that my PhD topic would involve phenomenology, chronic illness and other.

I was, at the time, working as a research assistant in the field of gastrointestinal disorders, and particularly, inflammatory bowel disease (IBD); this chronic, incurable relapsing-remitting auto-immune condition affects an estimated 500 000 people in the United Kingdom (HDRUK, 2020) and millions worldwide, especially in Westernised countries (Ng *et al.*, 2017). It is accompanied by several challenging symptoms, including fatigue, pain and urgency/incontinence. It was the latter that interested me: under the mentorship of Professor Christine Norton at King's College London, United Kingdom, I completed several studies addressing IBD-related incontinence (Dibley and Norton, 2013; Norton *et al.*, 2015; Dibley *et al.*, 2016); I had a growing insight into the shame, embarrassment and stigma experienced by many of those afflicted by this most antisocial of diseases. All of this – my fore-structures of understanding which comprised my personal history and the social influences as I grew up and entered adulthood, my being-in-the-world, my work as-researcher – combined to lead me towards the topic, and the research question, for my PhD: "*What is the experience of stigma in people with*

*Inflammatory bowel disease, with or without incontinence?"* This work showed forth a complex insight into participants' own fore-structures and how these influenced and, in some cases, mitigated against feelings of stigma (Dibley *et al.*, 2018).

## Thinking about stigma

One of the aspects of undertaking hermeneutic phenomenological research is the necessity of being in the research oneself; by acknowledging the temporal relationship we have with our world, and that our knowledge, understanding and perceptions are necessarily situated in and influenced by that world, we can embark on a journey of discovery with others. We can, with care, use our knowledge, prejudices, and the insights we already own on the path to further discovery, but we must not assume that we "know" the way. We need to be ready for surprising, unexpected, and often tantalising turns along our route. Thus, during analysis of my PhD data, I encountered a surprising phenomenon, but one which called loudly: alongside the well-documented, reported and researched forms of stigma, I saw hints of something subtly different – stigmatising attitudes and behaviours being directed towards the person with IBD by close family members. These insights directly challenged one of the concepts of the leading stigma theorist of the 20th century, Erving Goffman. Goffman's work, carried out in 1950s middle America, was based in symbolic interactionism (Blumer, 1986). By observing the micro-behaviours of ordinary interactions in everyday social settings, Goffman described how humans routinely yet diligently manage and control their behaviours with others in order to "fit in with the crowd" and give a good impression of self (Goffman, 1959). He then investigated the everydayness of those who did not fit in – the Others, leading to his seminal text on stigma (Goffman, 1963). Whilst Goffman has been criticised for outdated language, an oversimplified approach, and a lack of methodological detail (Burns, 1992; Sumner, 1994; Falk, 2001), his definition of stigma remains, in my view, widely applicable. Goffman describes stigma as *"an attribute that is deeply discrediting"* and that it is *"a language of relationships, not attributes, that is really needed"* (Goffman 1963, 12). This latter point is important: Goffman identifies, and others have since concurred, that it is not the attribute (the mark, the feature of difference) that is stigmatising, but that stigma arises from the relationships with observers, onlookers, witnesses and how they respond to that mark, or difference. Anything, from skin colour, to disability, to having a criminal record, to visible and invisible illnesses and more, may be stigmatising in some relationships and not others.

Since Goffman's work, numerous theorists have identified, labelled and presented various forms of stigma (Table 6.1), attaching a psychologically focussed ontic view, as if to say, stigma "is" this.

Reflecting on Goffman's assertion that stigma is relational, we start to appreciate an ontological view of stigma – its nature, its indefinable and situational qualities, the meaning it has to those who experience it. Classifying stigma in an ontic way ignores what it means to *feel* and *be* stigmatised, and the changeable

*Table 6.1* Types of stigma[1]

| Term | Meaning |
| --- | --- |
| Felt, self or internalised stigma | Internalised feelings of stigma; the individual stigmatises themselves independent of others' responses |
| Enacted, public or experienced stigma | Publics' (others') negative beliefs, feelings and behaviours expressed towards a person with a feature of difference; often seen as discrimination |
| Anticipated stigma | The expectation of being stigmatised by others |
| Perceived stigma | Believing oneself to be treated in a stigmatising way, even though this may not be the case |
| Courtesy stigma | Being stigmatised by association with someone who carries a feature of difference |

nature of that meaning according to the situation that a person might find them-selves in. For example, I do not feel stigmatised by my identity, but if I did, how could I measure it and say "My stigma 'is' this?" My experience of it would be very different if I were amongst a group of similarly identified women, of others with a variety of alternate identities, or of people who were, in every way, different to me. The ontic descriptions in Table 6.1 thus do not do justice to the existential qualities that are the focus of an ontological project using hermeneutic phenome-nology, where we are drawn into an exploration of what a given experience means and how those experiences are understood.

## The emergence of the kinship stigma study

Goffman considered that amongst the daily interactions of marked persons, there were two special relationships which afforded some protection against feeling stigmatised. He described these as the 'Own' (those with the same mark who have an allegiance of understanding) and the 'Wise' (those without the mark but whose special relationship with the person enables them to 'overlook' the mark and be supportive). For people with IBD, specialist clinicians and family members might be assumed to be 'The Wise' but what emerged from my PhD data, sug-gested otherwise.

Like other families, mine had skeletons in the cupboard. As I got older, I became increasingly aware of the efforts that family members, particularly my parents, employed to present a positive impression to the outside world. To all intents and purposes, we were an upper working-class family with a standard (for the time) structure of mother, father and two children, going about our business and contributing to the community through involvement with organisations such as Boy Scouts and Girl Guides, orchestras and church events. On the inside, it was very different. But my parents, I realised, had perfected the art of projecting an image of social normality and powerful social capital so effectively that it was never questioned. Naturally, then, when the hint of this family stigma emerged from my PhD, my interest was piqued. Once again, in a phenomenological way, everything that I was, that I understood, that I had learned and experienced in relation to this interesting phenomenon, surfaced for me and laid itself out as a path I had to follow. This then was my *"thrownness"* (Heidegger, 1962).

## Designing the project

As a developing hermeneutic scholar, I wanted to build on my PhD experiences by engaging in a methodological aspect that I had not yet enjoyed. A PhD is primarily a lone endeavour, although, in phenomenology studies, supervisors (including me) usually engage with "some" aspects of data analysis. Neither of my otherwise excellent supervisors was phenomenologists, and philosophical guidance was, therefore, unready-at-hand (and I noticed its absence) during my PhD studies. I now wanted to work with other hermeneutic scholars and benefit from their experience, particularly during data analysis. I invited colleagues from the Heideggerian Hermeneutic Institute in the United States, and was honoured to welcome Professor Tricia Young, Professor Pam Ironside, and Dr. Ellen Williams to my study team.

## Demonstrating the need for the study

The "hint" of the phenomenon, which I tentatively labelled as "kinship stigma" was not, by itself, enough to warrant investigation. I needed a sense of what had been done already, that the topic was sufficiently unique to pursue, and where the eventual findings would sit in relation to other literature. I conducted a systematic literature search (Dibley *et al.*, 2020) in which very few papers were located. One study on family stigma experienced by adult children caring for a parent with Alzheimer's disease (Werner *et al.*, 2010) reported courtesy stigma (see Table 6.1), which arose for participants due to their association with those whose condition is often stigmatised. Another (mixed-methods) study on adolescents with mental health problems explored their perceptions and experiences (but not meanings) of stigma originating from trusted others including family (Moses, 2010). These works only identified ontic descriptive understandings of stigma experienced or instigated by family members. I could find no hermeneutic phenomenological investigation of the topic. Family support is known to facilitate learning to live well with a chronic condition (Moskovitz *et al.*, 2000; Gallant, 2003; Altschuler *et al.*, 2009; Strom and Egede, 2012; Frohlich, 2014), and family is usually assumed to be supportive. We, therefore, sought to address the evidence gap through a hermeneutic phenomenological ontological inquiry into stigma instigated by family towards another family member.

## The research question

The structure of the research question is important to convey the philosophy, methodology and focus of the study. Since this was to be a hermeneutic phenomenological study, the research question was: *What is the experience and meaning of the social, emotional, and personal impact of kinship stigma in people with inflammatory bowel disease?* The word "experience" in this title indicates the project is ontological, and "meaning" highlights its interpretive focus; the core theme (kinship stigma) is identified, as are the areas of interest relating to this phenomenon (social, emotional and personal impact).

Although the "theme" of kinship stigma is stated in the question, we remained open to the possibility that this could change during the study, as the phenomenon – as understood and experienced by participants – revealed itself from the data. The research question is always just the starting point of hermeneutic inquiry as we hold ourselves open to the unbounded possibilities of ontological inquiry and what our question might reveal.

## Sample size

I am forever advising my MSc and PhD students delivering hermeneutic phenomenology studies that they should explain their sample size, not excuse it. The latter is an unhelpful yet lingering notion from the 1990s when qualitative methodologists were emerging amidst positivistic researchers and were still establishing robust arguments to demonstrate the credibility and trustworthiness of their work (and the language to describe it). Sample size in hermeneutic research is typically small but depends on many factors, including the rarity or sensitivity of the topic, the available population, and whether there are any sub-samples in the design. Other factors such as timescale and purpose (that is, educational qualification) are also influential. The aim, always, is to recruit enough people who can provide sufficient rich data with which to address the research question.

The kinship stigma study addressed a novel topic as it offered a counter-perspective to an assumed "supportive family relationship." Due to its methodological and philosophical approach, a wealth of rich data was expected. The lack of published evidence also suggested that it might be a reasonably rare experience, so the sample size was set at a minimum of 10. Offering an approximate rather than a specific number of participants permits flexibility (and avoids the need for an ethics amendment) should the need to gather more data arise – for instance, the emergence of an unexpected yet potentially important topic which warrants further investigation. To accommodate variety across the narratives, we interviewed 18 participants.

## Data collection

In hermeneutics, language is central to how we understand, make sense of, and share experiences. Addressing the hermeneutic relationship between speech and understanding, Gadamer (2003, p. 188) states that *"every act of understanding is … the inverse of an act of speech, the reconstruction of a construction."* We construct and reconstruct meaning through external dialogue with others and internal dialogue with our existing knowledge and understanding – the back and forth of conversation fuses with our internal yet silent active thinking as we seek to interpret what is being said – and brings us to a new point of understanding.

As humans, we do this naturally and subconsciously; we do not decide "to understand" – we are *always-already* "in the midst of what is, always listening and [already] responding" (Smythe *et al.*, 2008, 1396).

Techniques involving language that enable participants to tell their story as they understand it and in their own words are therefore philosophically necessary in hermeneutic phenomenological research. The hermeneutic "interview" is a dialogue: a spoken conversational exchange of ideas, opinions, or perceptions directed towards the exploration of a chosen subject. The purpose is to understand, rather than force an opinion or change the other participant's perspective. In hermeneutic phenomenology, the interview/conversation becomes a dialogue of understanding between data collector and participant, to co-create a "fusion of horizons" (Gadamer, 2003) as the new shared understanding is developed.

Our kinship stigma study, therefore, employed unstructured face-to-face individual interactions ("interview" is too formal a word) with participants who self-defined with a psychologically (ontically) orientated definition of stigma as *"being, or feeling that you are being treated differently and perhaps negatively, because of your IBD, by those close to you from whom you might expect to receive full support."* As is typical in hermeneutic phenomenological research, there was no pre-set or structured topic guide; this aspect can be challenging for novices presenting their studies for ethical review boards who require some evidence of how participants will be interviewed. The trick is to detail the trigger/opening/indicative questions, and give examples of prompts, and, crucially, to explain why this approach is methodologically sound. In the kinship stigma study, participants were invited to *"Tell me about a time when you felt stigmatised by a member of your family"* and follow up prompts and probes, such as *"You mentioned X, can you tell me more about that?"* ... and *"What did it mean to you when X happened?"* were guided by the participant's narrative.

All participants were UK residents, and I conducted all interactions. This decision was primarily pragmatic: a single data collector provided a degree of consistency and being in the same country as participants avoided the need to juggle time zones.

## Data analysis and findings

Data were analysed using a modification of Diekelmann and colleagues' (1989) guidance (see Dibley *et al.*, 2019) (a similar approach also undertaken by Bridget, Chapter 3). We conducted all team analysis sessions online and from the 235 single-spaced A4 pages of narrative data, three relational themes emerged: *Being Visible/Becoming Invisible*, *Being the disease/Having the disease*, and *Amplification, Loss and Suffering*, all woven together under the constitutive pattern: *Lacking Acknowledgement/Being Acknowledged*.

Overwhelmed with the richness and depth of the data and focussed on navigating our way to a meaningful representation of participants' experiences, we overlooked the potential presence of Heideggerian concepts in the findings. This does not mean that our initial analysis was flawed or "wrong" – but that further analysis would align this work with its philosophical underpinnings. The present chapter, therefore, provided a welcome opportunity to revisit and undertake a secondary analysis of that data.[2] Three of Heidegger's philosophical notions were revealed within participants' accounts: *pre-understanding*, *thrownness*, and *ready-at-hand/unready-at-hand*. There may, of course, be others, as the same data can be analysed through multiple lenses.

## Preunderstanding

According to Heidegger (1962), our preunderstanding (or fore-structures of under-standing) refers to fore-having (social, cultural and individual issues that exist already in our world before we come to understand them), fore-sight (what we are directed to pay attention to, based on our fore-having) and fore-conception (something we grasp, an opinion, bias, or meaning we ascribe, in advance). Our culture, the world we are born into, the social group we find ourselves in, our history and life experiences – all these aspects are already in our world before we come to know them, and before we come to think about them in relation to a particular experience. In a seminal text, Koch (1995, 831) explains that *"these stories are already within our common background understanding …pre-understanding is a structure of our 'being-in-the-world.' It is not something we can eliminate, or bracket, it is already with us in the world."* This is *fore-having*. Fore-having then influences *fore-sight*, which Heidegger describes as a definite decision to turn our sights towards understanding our fore-having, leading ultimately to *fore-understanding (or fore-conception)*, an interpretation of how this understanding should be conceived:

> Whenever something is interpreted as something, the interpretation will be founded essentially upon fore-having, fore-sight and fore-understanding.
>
> (Heidegger, 1962, 191)

These fore-structures give us a starting point and influence the way we perceive and understand the experiences we later find ourselves in.

In the kinship stigma study data, these fore-structures were expressed in the story of a young woman with ulcerative colitis, who experienced a flare up of her condition with acute abdominal pain and significant rectal bleeding on her wedding day:

> I think (my mum) genuinely thought I was exaggerating (about my illness), particularly on my actual wedding day. We were late because I couldn't get off the toilet because there was so much blood. And she just said it was nerves. And I was like, "Really, when you're nervous, do you have blood pouring out of you? Is that what happens, Mum?"
>
> (Dibley *et al.*, 2019, 1204)

Her mother not only attributed this outpouring to "wedding day nerves" but was more concerned about being late to the church than her daughter's wellbeing.

Later, afflicted by the fatigue that commonly occurs in IBD, the participant was not permitted to leave early and rest:

> The family wouldn't let me (leave) … 'People have come from miles, we've paid a fortune, make the most of it.'
>
> (Dibley *et al.*, 2019, 1205)

This data informed our "Lacking Acknowledgement/Being Acknowledged" constitutive pattern by highlighting the powerful influence of social norms and expectations that likely drove the family responses. However, it also constitutes Heidegger's fore-structures. The traditional social rules and expectations that pre-exist this woman's experience of her wedding are that the bride, arriving fashionably late, makes her grand entrance to eagerly waiting for guests. A lengthy delay creates anxieties for the groom, the officiating person, the bride's family, and the guests. The ceremony is followed by photographs, reception, speeches, party – a long and exhausting day in which the bride is expected to gleam and shine and be perpetually perfect. This is *fore-having* – the pre-existing cultural view of what a wedding is in Western cultures.

For those responsible for the planning and organising, there is a subtle and often unspoken pressure to "put on a good show," which creates, for them, a preliminary view of how the day should proceed. This is *fore-sight*. These two structures then influence the third: based on cultural rules (fore-having) and personal expectations (fore-sight), the family creates an understanding of what they must provide – not being late to the church, putting on a good show to reward people for the effort they have made to attend, and getting every last penny of value out of the money they have paid out to ensure guests have a good time. This is *fore-understanding* – the actual presentation of the wedding in the way that the family understand and believe their guests want to experience it. All of which can be anxiety-provoking, and by classifying her daughter's symptoms as anxiety, the mother doesn't have to consider the larger and potentially more problematic issue of her daughter being ill on this day of all days. These three Heideggerian structures – fore-having, fore-sight, and fore-understanding – help us appreciate the deeper meaning revealed by the family's behaviours.

## Thrownness

Heidegger's thinking on thrownness is complex (and also discussed by Polly, Chapter 3 and Lesley Kay in Chapter 5). It appears to present almost as a pre-destiny – we do not end up in the world we are in by accident or chance, but because of a history that precedes us and over which (particularly at the point of our birth) we have no control:

> As something thrown, Dasein has been thrown into existence. It exists as an entity which has to be as it is, and as it can be.
>
> (Heidegger, 1962, 321)

Withy (2014, 62) explains that *"we are thrown into something, delivered over to something, given over to something from which we have to start and with which we must deal."* For better or worse, the situation and context into which we are thrown at birth will, in some way, influence our path through life. Yet situatedness is not everything that Heidegger meant by thrownness. As Withy explains (2014, 66), something thrown travels *from* somewhere *to* somewhere else. This thrownness – our "landing" in a place, space and time – also sets us on a path such that our past is always before us. In other words, we travel the paths we do because of the paths we have already travelled – we are thrown forward to something because of where we are thrown from. Our historicity gives us a starting point such that we have somewhere or something that we come from, and this already determines where we go to. Heidegger explains the direction in which we travel as a "calling":

> The call is precisely something which *we ourselves* have neither planned nor prepared for nor voluntarily performed, nor have we ever done so. 'It' calls, against our expectations and even against our will. On the other hand, the call undoubtedly does not come from someone else who is with me in the world. The call comes *from* me and yet *from beyond me and over me* [emphasis in the original]
>
> (Heidegger, 1962, 320)

Thrownness also plays into our philosophical "travelling" – how and why we move from one point of understanding to another – how we attune ourselves to the daily experiences we find ourselves thrown into unexpectedly – sleeping through the alarm clock, getting a puncture in the car tyre, running out of milk. These are our micro journeys, where what we learn from past experiences gives us skills to attune ourselves to new experiences – to solve, to challenge, to question, to overcome, to adapt. Thrownness is a complex multifaceted concept involving many different ways of travelling through life.

In the kinship stigma study, thrownness was evident in May's experience of stigma from her sister and mother:

> Very soon after diagnosis, it kind of confirmed their view of me as somehow having caused it or created it or there was an inevitability about it, which led from damaged goods ... something broken and not quite right
>
> (Dibley *et al.*, 2019, 1203)

May had endured the unwanted attentions of her late abusive father. For her mother and sister, May's diagnosis of Crohn's disease in her early 20s was a direct consequence of her childhood experiences. For them, she was *thrown* forward into a damaged body and a life of chronic illness *from* a childhood that was damaged by abuse. May's mother and sister blamed her for the abuse and for the later illness, perceiving she had brought both forms of damage upon herself. Quite apart from the stigmatisation inherent in this attitude, it suggests a fatalistic view that there is nothing we can do to influence our thrownness. Superficially, we might consider the whence (where from) and wither (where to) of thrown-ness as irrefutable … we *will* end up where we end up *because of* our past, but this demands some intricate thinking. Whilst thrownness projects us towards a certain situation, we can make orientate to our new location by having a sense of "how" we arrived … in other words, we have a path that has taken us from where we came from, to where we now are … a sense of *"having-got-there-from-somewhere-else"* (Withy, 2014, 67) – in May's case, a traumatic and abusive past. It is also important to reflect that we can have agency on our path (albeit poten-tially curtailed by biopsychosocial and cultural factors) … so whilst thrownness projects us, we do have choices that we can make. We are constantly "thrown" into situations whereby a range of different possibilities and projections – different routes through – are possible.

For May's family, this intricate thinking is missing: their perception was "she came from bad – she's arrived at more bad" – but instead of acknowledging it sympathetically, they are critical of what they see as her failure to change the course of her life. Were it true that humans cannot influence their paths, no one would break out of poverty, no stories of "first in my family to attend univer-sity" would arise, and millions of people would not overcome childhood adversity. Thrownness is always informed by what has been and what is to come; it provides starting points and waypoints on our life course, but we can have influence by making choices.

## Ready-at-hand/unready-at-hand

At its simplest, Heidegger's thinking around ready-at-hand/unready-at-hand (or ready-to-hand/unready-to-hand) (also discussed by Bridget, Chapter 4) is a con-sideration of convenience and availability – an observation that the "things" we need in life are either readily available to us or not, and how our attention switches according to their availability. Of course, being Heidegger, it is not that simple … ready-at-hand and unready-at hand encompass the *mode* of the thing under consideration; a hammer, lying on the bench for the carpenter to use, is ready-at-hand because it is available, but this readiness-at-hand also includes the capacity of a hammer to be a hammer – which it becomes through the action involved in using it to hammer:

> The less we just stare at the hammer-thing, and the more we seize hold of it and use it, the more primordial does our relationship to it become, and the more unveiledly is it encountered as that which it is …
>
> (Heidegger, 1962, 98)

We can recognise a hammer by its constitutive features, but we also know it as a hammer when it functions as we expect it to. However, if the hammer is mislaid, breaks, or fails to function as expected, it becomes "unready-at-hand." This notion means that when something becomes unavailable to us, we really "notice" or consider the missing item in more authentic ways. The absent or broken hammer now sets us on a path of thinking with heightened awareness about how we will achieve our intended task without this core tool to help us – we thus begin to think more authentically about its purpose and our needs. Unready-at-hand is also termed "present-at-hand" – reflecting the change in our thinking from the unconscious (un-present – "ready-at-hand") to the conscious (presence) of heightened awareness of the object we are unable to use.

Can extend the thinking about these concepts beyond using them in relation to inanimate objects such as tools and equipment help us understand the meaning of experiences? Willerslev (2004) has applied the concept of ready-at-hand to spirits and dreaming, and Breivik (2010) – who also offers a nuanced interpretation of unready-at-hand as more than just unavailability – has addressed both in a detailed consideration of the experience of skydiving. Thomson (2011) uses these concepts in relation to women's conceptions of their body following a traumatic birth, and a PhD student of mine used it in relation to couples' infertility (Gale, unpublished PhD thesis). We can, then, also perhaps consider ready-at-hand/unready-at-hand in respect of people and of emotional support.

In the kinship stigma study, we see the expectation of ready-at-hand, and the distress of unready-at-hand, in the account of one participant who felt his parents were unavailable to him:

> It's the lack of support from something you came from. You're half of them— that's what it is. There should be more than just "I don't believe you!" Is that the best you can do? — It is a deeper feeling. It's somewhere down here in the gut. You need to be connected. The person with the disease needs to be accepted, especially from the parents. Without it, it's almost like an abandonment thing, I suppose.
>
> (Dibley *et al.*, 2019, 1205)

For this young man in his early 30s with ulcerative colitis, the emotional absence of his parents equated to being cast adrift – emotionally deserted and neglected – and left to deal with his situation alone. The expectation of readily available emotional support leads to an acute awareness and distress when it is unavailable – when it is unready-at-hand. We also see the role of expectation in respect of ready-at-hand and unready-at-hand in Simon's comments. His father had left the family home when Simon was a very young child and had never witnessed or experienced any of his son's illness which had been diagnosed after his departure:

> My mum and my dad are divorced. My dad lives in the Middle East. So, when I was ill, I never saw him, never heard from him. So that's good. But in terms of my mum, it was a, it was a bit difficult in the sense that whenever I was in hospital for treatment, which was pretty regularly the whole time, she's a teacher and she would always bring her coursework to the hospital with her. And I always felt guilty that I was pulling her away from work or that she had other things to be doing. (Unpublished study data)

Simon dismisses his father's absence with "so that's good" –his father had never been ready-at-hand and wasn't expected to be, but his response to his mother is different. His mother was both ready-at-hand by being physically present but unready-at-hand due to not being emotionally connected with or focussing on her son. He always felt she "*had other things to be doing.*"

The impact of family being unready-at-hand – unavailable or not offering support as expected – is profound. We may not think about the unconditional "ready-to-hand" love and support within our important and intimate relationships if what they provide is consistent – it is just "there," available whenever we need it. It only becomes noticeable in its absence – and then all we see is what is not there. The absence thus becomes "present at hand" – taking front stage in our consciousness as we think and reflect on what this absence means to us. In our study, parental "unready-at-hand" was interpreted and understood by participants as stigmatising.

## The joys, challenges and pitfalls of undertaking hermeneutic phenomenological research

Delivering hermeneutic phenomenological research is both a joy and a challenge. Engaging with a research methodology that "sits comfortably" with me enables deep exploration of human experiences in the world, celebrates and values my connectedness with the subjects I explore, and provides a philosophical, theoretical, and practical challenge which continues to inspire and motivate me, is a joy. I like that it is not easy, that it invites me to think deeply and authentically – that it hands me a responsibility to authentically foreground the voices of participants. It is what Smythe and Spence (2019, 7) describe as "*the gift of the struggle.*" Working with others in a hermeneutic team is uplifting, inspiring and encouraging: a well-chosen team creates a safe environment in which to acknowledge one's own biases, weaknesses and prejudices – and from which new insights, paths and adventures unfold. We are always "on the way towards" something – a new insight, realisation, awareness and understanding of our own self – as well as journeying towards addressing the research question.

The biggest challenges for me lie in data collection and analysis. Engaging others in conversation is easy enough but engaging them in a hermeneutic manner is a different thing entirely. It took me ages to learn the art of hermeneutic interviewing – of pointing participants towards a phenomenon of interest and creating the space for them to explore that at their own pace – my enthusiasm often (especially in early years) led me to talk too much, guide too closely, jump in with my assumed understandings. At the Hermeneutic Institute in the United States, I recall being invited by Pam Ironside and Sherrie Sims to "demonstrate" the art of interviewing. I was to interview Sherrie whilst my peers observed. I thought I was helping to teach them (and there was probably an element of that), but on reflection, it taught me so much more. Sherrie didn't play ball, and the dialogue brilliantly and expertly demonstrated how easy it is to fall into non-hermeneutic traps. It completely changed my way of interviewing, and now I "have" it, I find it difficult to do it any other way. Reverting to standard approaches when I am invited to add my qualitative experience to other non-phenomenological studies becomes its own challenge – I always want to know more, to explore further, even though the study may not require that. It is difficult to not be phenomenological when it is fundamental to one's own being. Collecting data is as much about what you do say as what keeps you silent. Enthusiasm can cause one to leap ahead (take over) by blurting out the thinking going on in one's head instead of waiting patiently, giving the participant time, and creating the space for them to (more often than not) verbalise the very thing that is showing up for you, desperate to be released. Technique, and patience, challenge me constantly.

I love doing data analysis –the processes of working with others, of combining thinking, of generating early ideas together and seeing those grow, move and reshape organically. I love the moments when someone tentatively offers an emerging idea, and everyone else has "seen" the same thing. The excitement and sense of honesty towards the kinship stigma study data that emerged when we realised, we had all settled on one single powerful image was extraordinary.

Yet, at the same time, data analysis is challenging. I do not mind that it is time-consuming, but it can be very difficult to find the time – not just to work with the data, but to think. I always advise my students to schedule in more time for analysis than they usually think they'll need – because to do it well means not rushing. Time is needed – time to think, dwell, sit with the data, to allow oneself not to try too hard – and in relaxing, to trust that meaning will show itself. Fitting that into a busy schedule is not easy.

A related challenge is to know when data analysis is "done," though perhaps a better phrase would be "done enough." Analysis can never be claimed to be complete because you can never "know" that you have seen and understood all the data could offer – but we need to be able to demonstrate thoroughness in our hermeneutic processes. For me, a sure sign that data analysis is not "done enough" is when I am unsettled with things as they are, and the data is still invading my thinking because there are still things to be thought about. I learnt – from Nancy Diekelmann – to expect loose ends because experiences, and the data arising from them, are not neat packages. Yet having a coherent shape to the data – and thus to the experience – is a pre-requisite to describing that experience to others. If the data are still "messy" and I cannot visualise the shape of it clearly, then it is not "done enough."

Pitfalls can mostly be avoided by careful planning, by ensuring a solid relationship between philosophy, methodology and method so that at all stages, rationale can be given for what was done, and why, and the study can be reported robustly. Careful attention to detail in the selection of participants, collection and analysis of data, reflexivity and management of self predisposes to a smoother study experience and transition to publication. Diligent record-keeping is also important – for example, labelling data extracts in preparation for analysis enables an easy return to the original transcript to relocate key quotes, whenever necessary.

## Final reflections

Doing hermeneutic phenomenological research means carrying Heidegger along with us through all phases of our project and – where and when appropriate – using his thoughts to help reveal insight and meaning in the data. Heidegger is not the only way of revealing meaning, but where his work can add insight, offer another way of understanding, or augment the contribution of extant literature, it should be used. Doing so adds authenticity to our work.

Thinking about Heidegger's philosophy and the research methodology that is hermeneutic phenomenology brings me to the point of realisation: I feel "at home" with it all. Jacobson explains this perfectly when she writes that:

> being-at-home is essentially an experience of passivity [but] … also a way of being *to which we attain*. In other words, we are active in our being passive: we are beings whose experience of home is that of an *essential* and *inherent* background and foundation, but this foundation has been *developed* through our very efforts of *learning* how to dwell.
>
> (Jacobson, 2009, 356, emphasis in the original)

I feel both passively and actively comfortable at home with Heidegger; it is where my own spirit and way of being-in-the-world feel welcome and as though it belongs. There is space here for me to be unique, to be different, and I am happy that this is where – philosophically – I dwell. Yet I have also had to learn *how* to dwell – how to make space for thinking, to open myself to the possibility of other, and to embrace, explore and understand. Hermeneutic phenomenology gives me the space I need to think and to consider, welcome and respect any number of other possible explanations and interpretations. And in thinking, I find myself, my focus, and my way of dwelling.

## Notes

1. It is important to note that Goffman didn't label these themes/ideas and meanings – it appears others have done that since. Although these labels are credited to his body of works, no one really seems to know who to credit for each label.
2. Secondary analysis of data collected in hermeneutic phenomenology studies is not problematic because there is no such thing as one meaning or one truth. Other interpretations will always surface from the same experience when a new reader with a different gaze casts their eye – and this can challenge the novice hermeneutic researcher hoping to present the final and complete "interpretation" of their data. I urge the novice to relax – there can never be a definitive interpretation, only what you – at this moment in time and space – see and understand in your participants' experiences.

## References

Altschuler, A. *et al.* (2009) "The influence of husbands' or male partners' support on women's psychosocial adjustment to having an ostomy resulting from colorectal cancer," *Journal of Wound, Ostomy and Continence Nursing*, 36(3), pp. 299–305. doi: 10.1097/WON.0b013e3181a1a1dc.

Blumer, H. (1986) *Symbolic Interactionism: Perspective and Method.* Reprint. Berkeley, CA: University of California Press.

Breivik, G. (2010) "Being-in-the-void: A Heideggerian analysis of skydiving," *Journal of the Philosophy of Sport*, 37(1), pp. 29–46. doi: 10.1080/00948705.2010.9714764.

Burns, T. (1992) *Erving Goffman.* London: Routledge.

Canales, M. K. (2000) "Othering: Toward an understanding of difference," *Advances in Nursing Science.* Lippincott Williams and Wilkins, 22(4), pp. 16–31. doi: 10.1097/00012272-200006000-00003.

Carpenter, M. (2018) "The 'normalization' of intersex bodies and 'othering' of intersex identities in Australia," *Journal of Bioethical Inquiry.* Springer Netherlands, pp. 487–495. doi: 10.1007/s11673-018-9855-8.

Dibley, L. (2009) "Experiences of lesbian parents in the UK: Interactions with midwives," *Evidence based Midwifery*, 7, pp. 94–100.

Dibley, L. *et al.* (2016) "Development and initial validation of a disease-specific bowel continence questionnaire for inflammatory bowel disease patients," *European Journal of Gastroenterology & Hepatology.* Lippincott Williams and Wilkins, 28(2), pp. 233–239. doi: 10.1097/MEG.0000000000000513.

Dibley, L. *et al.* (2020) *Doing Hermeneutic Phenomenological Research: A Practical Guide.* London: Sage Publications.

Dibley, L. and Norton, C. (2013) "Experiences of fecal incontinence in people with inflammatory bowel disease: Self-reported experiences among a community sample," *Inflammatory Bowel Diseases*, 19(7), pp. 1450–1462. doi: 10.1097/MIB.0b013e318281327f.

Dibley, L., Norton, C. and Whitehead, E. (2018) "The experience of stigma in inflammatory bowel disease: An interpretive (hermeneutic) phenomenological study," *Journal of Advanced Nursing*, 74(4), pp. 838–851. doi: 10.1111/jan.13492.

Dibley, L., Williams, E. and Young, P. (2019) "When family don't acknowledge: A hermeneutic study of the experience of kinship stigma in community-dwelling people with inflammatory bowel disease," *Qualitative Health Research.* SAGE Publications, Inc., p. 1049732319831795. doi: 10.1177/1049732319831795.

Diekelmann, N. L. *et al.* (1989) *The NLN Criteria for Appraisal of Baccalaureate Programs : A Critical Hermeneutic Analysis.* New York: National League for Nursing.

Falk, G. (2001) *Stigma: How We Treat Outsiders.* Amherst, NY: Prometheus Books.

Foshay, T. (1999) "Intentionality, originarity, and the "Always Already" in Derrida and Gans – Anthropoetics IV, no. 1 Spring/Summer 1999: *Special Issue on Deconstruction, Anthropoetics: The Journal of Generative Anthropology.* Available at: http://anthropoetics. ucla.edu/ap0401/foshay/ (Accessed: 18 June 2021).

Frohlich, D. O. (2014) "Support often outweighs stigma for people with inflammatory bowel disease," *Gastroenterology Nursing*, 37(2). Available at: https://journals. lww.com/gastroenterologynursing/Fulltext/2014/03000/Support_Often_Outweighs_ Stigma_for_People_With.2.aspx.

Gadamer, H. (2003) *Truth and Method* (transl. J. Weinsheimer and D. G. Marshall). 2nd revised edn. London: Continuum.

Gallant, M. P. (2003) "The influence of social support on chronic illness self-management: A review and directions for research," *Health Education and Behavior.* SAGE Publications, pp. 170–195. doi: 10.1177/1090198102251030.

Goffman, E. (1959) *The Presentation of Self in Everyday Life.* Woodstock, NY: Overlook Press.

Goffman, E. (1963) *Stigma : Notes on the Management of Spoiled Identity.* Englewood Cliffs, NJ: Prentice-Hall.

HDRUK (2020) *Gut Reaction – The Health Data Research Hub for Inflammatory Bowel Disease – HDR UK*. Available at: https://www.hdruk.ac.uk/help-with-your-data/our-hubs-across-the-uk/gut-reaction/ (Accessed: 9 October 2020).

Heidegger, M. (1962) *Being and Time* (transl. J. Macquarrie & E. Robinson). New York: Harper Perennial.

Heidegger, M. (1971) *On the Way to Language* (transl. P. D. Hertz). New York, NY: Harper & Row.

Jacobson, K. (2009) "A developed nature: A phenomenological account of the experience of home," *Continental Philosophy Review*, 42, pp. 355–373. doi: 10.1007/s11007-009-9113-1.

Johnson, J. L. *et al.* (2004) "Othering and being othered in the context of health care services," *Health Communication*. Routledge, 16(2), pp. 255–271. doi: 10.1207/s15327027hc1602_7.

Koch, T. (1995) "Interpretive approaches in nursing research: The influence of Husserl and Heidegger," *Journal of Advanced Nursing*. John Wiley & Sons Ltd, 21(5), pp. 827–836. doi: 10.1046/j.1365-2648.1995.21050827.x.

McCann, C. and Kim, S.-K. (2003) *Feminist Theory Reader: Local and Global Perspectives*. New York, NY: Routledge.

Moses, T. (2010) "Being treated differently: Stigma experiences with family, peers, and school staff among adolescents with mental health disorders," *Social Science and Medicine*, 70(7), pp. 985–993. doi: 10.1016/j.socscimed.2009.12.022.

Moskovitz, D. N. *et al.* (2000) "Coping behavior and social support contribute independently to quality of life after surgery for inflammatory bowel disease," *Diseases of the Colon and Rectum*, 43(4), pp. 517–521. doi: 10.1007/BF02237197.

Ng, S. C. *et al.* (2017) "Worldwide incidence and prevalence of inflammatory bowel disease in the 21st century: A systematic review of population-based studies," *The Lancet*. Lancet Publishing Group, 390(10114), pp. 2769–2778. doi: 10.1016/S0140-6736(17)32448-0.

Norton, C. *et al.* (2015) "Faecal incontinence intervention study (FINS): Self-management booklet information with or without nurse support to improve continence in people with inflammatory bowel disease: Study protocol for a randomized controlled trial," *Trials*, 16(1). doi: 10.1186/s13063-015-0962-0.

Petros, G. *et al.* (2006) "HIV/AIDS 'othering' in South Africa: The blame goes on," *Culture, Health and Sexuality*. Cult Health Sex, 8(1), pp. 67–77. doi: 10.1080/13691050500391489.

Smythe, E. A. *et al.* (2008) "Doing Heideggerian hermeneutic research: A discussion paper," *International Journal of Nursing Studies*, 45(9), pp. 1389–1397. https://doi.org/10.1016/j.ijnurstu.2007.09.005.

Smythe, E. and Spence, D. (2019) "Reading Heidegger," *Nursing Philosophy*. doi: 10.1111/nup.12271.

Stenstad, G. (2006) *Transformations: Thinking after Heidegger*. Madison, WI: University of Wisconsin Press.

Strom, J. L. and Egede, L. E. (2012) "The Impact of social support on outcomes in adult patients with type 2 diabetes: A systematic review," *Current Diabetes Reports*. NIH Public Access, pp. 769–781. doi: 10.1007/s11892-012-0317-0.

Sumner, C. (1994) *The Sociology of Deviance: An Obituary*. Buckingham: Open University Press.

Thomson, G. (2011) "Abandonment of Being in childbirth." In *Qualitative Research in Midwifery and Childbirth: Phenomenological Approaches*, edited by G. Thomson, F. Dykes and S. Downe, 133–152. London: Routledge.

Werner, P., Goldstein, D. and Buchbinder, E. (2010) "Subjective experience of family stigma as reported by children of Alzheimer's disease patients," *Qualitative Health Research*. SAGE Publications, 20(2), pp. 159–169. doi: 10.1177/1049732309358330.

Willerslev, R. (2004) "Spirits as 'ready to hand': A phenomenological analysis of Yukaghir spiritual knowledge and dreaming," *Anthropological Theory*. SAGE Publications, 4(4), pp. 395–418. doi: 10.1177/1463499604047918.

Withy, K. (2014) "Situation and limitation: Making sense of Heidegger on thrownness," *European Journal of Philosophy*. Blackwell Publishing Ltd, 22(1), pp. 61–81. doi: 10.1111/j.1468-0378.2011.00471.x.

Young-Bruehl, E. (1996) *The Anatomy of Prejudice*. Cambridge, MA: Harvard University Press.

# 7 Embodied hermeneutic phenomenology

## Bringing the lived body into health professions education research

*Helen F. Harrison and Elizabeth Anne Kinsella*

### Abstract

In this chapter, we propose that hermeneutic phenomenology can be enriched through deeper attention to embodiment and embodied perspectives. French philosopher Maurice Merleau-Ponty's philosophical insights on embodiment, intersubjectivity and intercorporeality, as well as insights from other thinkers who focus on embodiment, are invoked to inform an embodied hermeneutic phenomenological methodology. The application of this approach – and the contributions to knowledge that it can offer – are considered drawing on examples from a study of student peer mentorship in nursing education. The ways in which an embodied perspective can shape various aspects of research are highlighted. The aim is to make visible what an embodied hermeneutic phenomenological methodology might look like in research in health- and social-care contexts. In this chapter, we describe the theoretical foundations of this approach, discuss the ways in which these perspectives underpinned the design and analysis of a health professions education research project, and provide specific examples of foregrounding embodied perspectives in our research questions, methods and data analysis.

## Embodied hermeneutic phenomenology

The impetus for an embodied hermeneutic phenomenological approach to study peer mentorship arose from a constellation of research interests, theoretical perspectives and practical educational experiences. Helen Harrison is a college nursing professor in a collaborative nursing degree program in Southwestern Ontario. In her early years, she developed a curiosity about the workings of the human body; her father shared his belief that our bodies contributed to thinking and wrote about his idea that unconscious thoughts and actions originate from the body (Gooding, 1968). Elizabeth Anne Kinsella is a scholar of health professions education and practice, with interest in reflective practice, embodiment, and professional knowledge. She is a qualitative researcher interested in hermeneutic phenomenology, the hermeneutics of the visual and arts-based approaches to knowledge generation.

In Helen's observations with nursing students in a peer mentorship program that she facilitates, she noticed that students related to each other differently than with faculty, in a way that might be described as more embodied. Reflecting

DOI: 10.4324/9781003081661-7

on this gave birth to an interest in bringing an embodied lens to peer membership programs in health professional education. Studying and writing about Maurice Merleau-Ponty's work on embodiment (Harrison et al., 2019) laid the foundation for an embodied hermeneutic phenomenological approach to research. The aim of the study was to contribute to knowledge about student peer mentors' cognitive and embodied perceptions of teaching and learning in a Canadian undergraduate nursing program.

Peer mentorship is on the rise in nursing and other health professions education programs in many areas of the world, including North America, Australia, Turkey and the United Kingdom (Andersen and Watkins, 2018). Student-peer mentors are students within the same program who help other students to develop professional capabilities over at least one academic term (McKenna and Williams, 2017). Given decreased availability of clinical practice sites, professional skills are increasingly being practiced in lab or simulation settings. This has resulted in a need for greater support of students in the lab and more calls for peer mentorship programs (Ramm et al., 2015). We wanted to understand students' experiences of peer mentorship and how it shaped the learning experiences of peer mentors and mentees. Additionally, we wanted to find a way to attend to not only students' cognitive perceptions but also their embodied perceptions.

We reasoned that hermeneutic phenomenology would be a fruitful methodological approach for this research due to its focus on meanings and relationships in context and its interpretive, dialogic and reflexive nature (Gadamer, 1960/1975; Dowling, 2007; Kinsella and Bidinosti, 2015). We were also intrigued by the powerful insights about embodiment being put forward in Merleau-Ponty's phenomenological writings. Nonetheless, it was surprising to find few methodological resources that integrated an explicit focus on embodied perspectives within hermeneutic phenomenology. In response, we set out to articulate a research approach that would allow for exploration of participants' embodied knowledge through what we propose as an "embodied hermeneutic phenomenological methodology."

This journey to an embodied methodological approach was not a straight path. In many ways, it felt as if this approach "chose us." We were interested in practice scholarship, where a number of scholars contend that a significant amount of professional knowledge is embodied (Green, 2015; Kinsella, 2009), and we were particularly interested in theoretical perspectives that could help illuminate embodied perspectives. Most theories of embodiment point to the writings of Merleau-Ponty, which led us to an exploration of his writing, particularly focused on embodiment, intersubjectivity and intercorporeality. (Harrison et al., 2019). Merleau-Ponty argues for recognition of the body as a means of perception; we were intrigued to explore what his philosophical insights might offer to research focused on embodied learning. We were challenged with how to honour knowledge arising through the body without filtering that knowledge through a solely cognitive process, and we were interested in questions concerning how to convey embodied knowledge to others in the context of student peer mentorship in nursing.[1]

## Dwelling with Merleau-Ponty: Embodiment, intersubjectivity, and intercorporeality

We spent time dwelling in Merleau-Ponty's philosophical writings on embodiment, intersubjectivity, and intercorporeality (Harrison et al., 2019), which informs our "embodied" hermeneutic phenomenological methodology. A summary of these three key philosophical ideas is outlined below.

*Embodiment:* Much of Merleau-Ponty's philosophical work is written with a view of human knowledge as embodied. He highlights the primacy of the body as an instrument for understanding the world:

> My body is the … very actuality of the phenomenon of expression … it is the common texture of all objects and is, at least with regard to the perceived world, the general instrument of my understanding.
>
> (Merleau-Ponty, 2012, 244)

Recognising the body as a means of perception was a fundamental orientation informing our research design. We wanted to access knowledge experienced through the body, for example, the sinking feeling in the gut when an upsetting situation arises or the bodily sense that someone in our presence is in distress.

Merleau-Ponty draws on principles of *Gestalt* theory[2] to show that the figure of attention stands out against a background during perception – recognising that there may be differing aspects of phenomena that are foregrounded at the same time by different people, shaped in part by each person's embodied perceptions. These ideas are generative for researchers to recognise that one's embodiment shapes perception, and may be different for individual researchers and participants, despite shared aims to investigate a phenomenon. For example, a researcher may espouse goals relating to enhancing understanding of the experience of peer mentorship. A participant, on the other hand, may wish to enhance the mentorship program as their main priority. There may also be varying aspects that different researchers foreground and background within the same project, or that different students' foreground and background – like a mosaic that is constantly shifting. For example, research teams with members from different health disciplines may bring distinctly nuanced perspectives that foreground and background different aspects of teaching and learning or of student-client interactions. This may create epistemic tensions and/or enrich interpretations of data. Relatedly, Merleau-Ponty writes about embodied style. He says, along with existence, "*I received a way of existing, or a style. All of my actions and thoughts are related to the structure*" of this embodied style (2012, 482). This idea is useful for identifying different embodied styles of phenomena. For instance, we asked participants about their styles of being a peer mentor and observed their embodied styles of interacting with mentees during participant observation.

*Intersubjectivity:* Merleau-Ponty was also interested in intersubjectivity. He wrote about the social world as a "*permanent field of existence*" (379). Another way of wording this is to say that world is "*always already social*". One way in which attention to intersubjectivity was foregrounded in our study was through attention to collaborative interpretive processes in the data collection design and approach to analysis. Merleau-Ponty considers dialogue between two people as a condition for constituting common ground. He wrote

> in the experience of dialogue, a common ground is constituted between me and another; my thoughts and his (*sic*) form a single fabric … a shared operation of which neither of us is the creator. Here there is a being-shared-by-two. (2012, 370)

This is similar to what is gestured by Gadamer's (1975) idea of a " fusion of horizons" whereby two interlocutors[3] come to a common understanding through dialogue. When considering this type of collaborative meaning-making between researcher/ professor and student in collecting and analysing data, it is important to reflexively consider how power differentials may shape the nature of the interactions (Guenther, 2019). Bearing this in mind, we contend that Merleau-Ponty's ideas about reciprocal contributions through dialogue and the possibility that our words and those of others become a "shared operation" of sorts, a "single fabric" in which the whole is greater than the sum of its parts, are fruitful insights for embodied research design. An example of these ideas is provided later in the analysis section.

*Intercorporeality:* Merleau-Ponty also foregrounds intercorporeality. Intercorporeality attends to the ways in which people attune to the bodies of others. Merleau-Ponty writes

> My two hands 'coexist' or are 'compresent' because they are one single body's hands. The other person appears through an extension of that compresence." Merleau-Ponty goes on to say, "he and I are like organs of one single intercorporeality. (1964, 168)

When two bodies come together as intercorporeal beings, Merleau-Ponty suggests that the subject's intentions " inhabit" the body of the other. This is not to say that one understands another as well as one understands oneself, but rather that:

> Communication or the understanding of gestures is achieved through the reciprocity between my intentions and the other person's gestures, and between my gestures and the intentions which can be read in the other person's behavior. Everything happens as if the other person's intention inhabited my body, or as if my intentions inhabited his body.
>
> (Merleau-Ponty, 2012, 190–191)

Reciprocity speaks to a two-way process. This passage refers to a persons' intentions as communicated through gestures. For Merleau-Ponty, even speech is a gesture, it is embodied and occurs between individuals and, as such, represents an intercorporeal process. Other gestures of communication include movements of the body such as hand gestures and facial expressions, which have meaning within

*Table 7.1* Towards an embodied hermeneutic

| Characteristics of hermeneutics (Kinsella, 2006) | Characteristics of hermeneutics: infused with insights from Merleau-Ponty (Harrison et al., 2019) |
|---|---|
| 1. Seeks understanding rather than explanation | 1. The hermeneutic quest for "understanding" comes through the body – moving beyond language and cognition – to include understanding that arises through embodied being in the world |
| 2. Acknowledges the situated location of interpretation | 2. The location of interpretation is situated within intersubjective relationships among researchers and participants |
| 3. Recognises the role of language and historicity in interpretation | 3. Attending to participants' evocative wording and embodied language and responses |
| 4. Views inquiry as conversation | 4. Given assumptions about the body's role in communication through dialogue among embodied participants, intercorporeality is foregrounded in interpretive acts |
| 5. Comfortable with ambiguities | 5. The aim is not to develop "essences" or "truths" but rather to foreground diverse perspectives |

a shared culture (Cuffari and Streeck, 2017). Across cultures, specific gestures can have different and even opposite meanings. When people from different cultures interact, therefore, clarification may be needed, as it is not only two individuals but also two cultures that come into communication. Differing meanings of gestures may also occur in communication between different generations, such as between a young-adult student and a middle-aged professor/researcher. Since peer mentorship activities and research activities involve intercorporeal gestures and communication, Merleau-Ponty's ideas shaped our research design and informed our reflexive attention throughout the peer mentorship study.

In the following sections, we show how the theoretical perspectives of embodiment, intersubjectivity and intercorporeality are fruitful for embodied approaches to hermeneutic phenomenology.

### Embodiment and hermeneutics

Kinsella's (2006) articulation of hermeneutics in qualitative research, which drew on Gadamer (1975) and other hermeneutic thinkers, was our starting point. We incorporated these characteristics of hermeneutics with insights from Merleau-Ponty's work (Harrison et al., 2019) to articulate an embodied hermeneutic (see Table 7.1).

### Embodiment and phenomenology

Given phenomenology's philosophical foundations, using it to ground empirical research can present challenges. For example, it may be impossible to capture "unreflected" experience due to the research process occurring retrospective of experience; nonetheless, in the peer mentor study, we endeavoured to encourage the most immediate participant descriptions possible. One strategy was not to reveal interview questions to participants in advance. The hope was to evoke fresh, raw, spontaneous, pre-conceptual descriptions that move beyond intentional cognitive reflection and in this way, elicit more embodied responses (Kinsella, 2012; Harrison, 2021).

Eugene Gendlin (1962, 1981), a philosopher and psychologist, theorised about the role of the body in creating meaning, drawing on Merleau-Ponty's ideas. Gendlin considers the phenomenon of "preconceptual experiencing" as *"raw, present, ongoing functioning (in us) of what is usually called experience"*; he describes it as a concretely present flow of feeling for which, *"at any moment, we can individually and privately direct our attention inward … and there it is … we can put only a few aspects of it into words … our definitions, our knowing 'what it is', are symbols that specify aspects of it, 'parts' of it"* (1962, 11).

This attention to bodily felt meaning, or bodily felt sense, informed data collection in our study. Participants were encouraged to access their felt sense when responding to both speech-based and arts-based research methods, and to create phrases, images and symbols, to accompany verbal accounts of these symbols and words. The specific instructions to participants and some of their resulting responses are highlighted in a later section.

## Embodied methods

We drew on theoretical perspectives from Merleau-Ponty to underpin the methods of the study, which were designed to purposefully elicit embodied perspectives. This included a focus on embodied perception, the design of research questions, interview questions, body mapping and reflexivity.

Embodied Research Questions:

The question of how to develop phenomenological research questions informed by theories of embodiment is a challenge. In our study, we brought explicit attention to embodied perceptions in the articulation of our research questions:

What are students' cognitive/embodied perceptions of teaching and learning through peer mentorship within a BScN education program?

What are students' cognitive/embodied perceptions of peer mentorship relationships within this program?

What meanings and embodied understandings are revealed about peer mentorship through words, images and symbols created during a body mapping process?

## Embodied interview questions

Next, we designed an interview guide that elicits embodied perceptions. We used Merleau-Ponty's work to ground 5 of 12 interview questions, and Lakoff and Johnson (2008), Samuel Mallin (1996) and Gendlin (1962) to inform 2 further

*Table 7.2* Embodied hermeneutic phenomenological interview questions

| Embodied perspective | Author | Interview questions |
| --- | --- | --- |
| Figure against background | Merleau-Ponty (2012) | What stands out for you about your experience of the peer mentorship program? |
| Embodiment | Merleau-Ponty (2012) | Can you think of any experiences related to the body that stand out in peer mentorship?<br>Probes:<br>• [any] embodied perceptions or responses (chill up the spine? sinking feeling in the gut? etc.?)<br>• senses such as smells, sounds, sights or tactile feelings?<br>• nonverbal forms of communication?<br>• positionality of bodies in the lab? |
| Style | Merleau-Ponty (2012) | Tell me about your "style" of being a peer mentor. |
| Intersubjectivity | Merleau-Ponty (2012) | Can you speak to the nature of the relationships you've experienced within the program? |
| Intercorporeality | Merleau-Ponty (2012) | Tell me about your awareness of your or your mentee's bodies in space or in relation during peer mentorship activities. |
| Metaphor | Lakoff and Johnson (2008)<br>Gendlin (1962) | If you were to create a metaphor to represent your experience in the peer mentorship program, what might it be? |
| Images | Samuel Mallin (1996) | If you were to create an image to represent your experience in the peer mentorship program, what might it be? |

questions that use metaphor and image to invoke embodied understandings (see Table 7.2). Below are examples of 7 of 12 interview questions explicitly informed by embodied perspectives.

During the pilot testing process for the interview guide, it came to light that a smoother transition between discussing general aspects of teaching and learning and those directly involving the body was needed. Questions related to embodied responses seemed to take participants by surprise. To smooth the transition from more "cognitive" to more "embodied" questions, we acknowledged our interest in embodied aspects of peer mentorship and let participants know that the next few questions would be related to bodily experiences. We were intentional about nurturing Merleau-Ponty's insights about dialogue, asking probing questions to approach mutual understanding about what participants were expressing verbally and with bodily gestures – Helen asked participants to confirm the interpretations of meaning at the moment if there seemed to be ambiguity.

## Embodied interview data: Exemplars

The interview questions enabled us to elicit embodied responses; here are exemplars of how embodiment was revealed in the interview data.

*Exemplar 1:*   When asked about bodily responses during mentorship activities, James shared the pride and happiness that stood out for him:

*Respondent (R):*   I feel like that swelling sense of pride that just surges through you, like the overwhelming happiness, almost, like when you are just excited when students are learning. When you see them have those moments where they are like, oh, I've got it, that is deeply an embodied sensation that is very satisfying … to experience.

*Moderator (M):*   You are feeling it inside you?

*R:*   Yes.

*M:*   In a particular place?

*R:*   You just feel it in your chest, kind of. You're almost like taking a deep breath and … it's like a sigh, like they got it, that's good, something like that.

*Exemplar 2:*   Emma recalled her embodied responses while interacting with her mentees in the lab, including observing their manner with standardised patients[4] and during conversations about what mentees were struggling with:

> Sometimes, when I would see first year students treat the [standardized patients] poorly, it sent a chill up my spine: Ooh, either you improve your bedside manner a lot, or that's going to probably end up being your nursing. … I guess there was always a little bit of pressure in your gut, that you were telling them the wrong information, or guiding them in the wrong direction. Then again, when they confide in you, and they're crying, or if they're talking about their struggles outside of school … one student was taking care of a dying (family member) … It was just so intense … I don't know where that is in the body, I know it hurts my heart when I hear those things, but it's a little bit of a sinking feeling because you can't do much … you're pretty much just listening … those are the feelings that I felt.

## Embodiment and body mapping method

Body mapping is an emergent method that researchers contend can access embodied forms of knowledge (de Jager et al., 2016; Gastaldo et al., 2012; Solomon, 2002). Body mapping was a second method used in the peer mentor study. Body mapping involves drawing visual representations of bodily responses to guided questions. This approach foregrounds the body in generating meaning and assists participants to describe personal journeys of learning through time (McCorquodale and DeLuca, 2020; Orchard, 2017). Body mapping involves:

> Using drawing, painting or other art-based techniques to visually represent aspects of people's lives, their bodies and the world they live in. Body

mapping is a way of telling stories, much like totems that contain symbols with different meanings, but whose significance can only be understood in relation to the creator's overall story and experience.

(Gastaldo et al., 2012, 5)

Visual and arts-based methods such as body maps have the potential to engage embodied meanings in ways that move beyond cognitive and language-based approaches (Davey, 1999). Body mapping method shares aspects of phenomenology, narrative reasoning, arts-based research, and participatory research methods (McCorquodale and DeLuca, 2020). It provides a central representational space for the body, encouraging participants to *"engage in a conversation about experience and perceptions as lived in an embodied manner, rather than in a temporal or spatial way"* (Gastaldo et al., 2012, 11).

Jane Solomon describes body mapping as a method that inquires into *"everything that we feel is most important about ourselves"*; it helps people *"to get a better understanding about themselves, their bodies and the world they live in"* (2002, 2). She goes on to say that body mapping can reach out to people *"in social and political ways"* (3). Guided body-mapping questions and an example of a participant body map from the current study are presented later in the chapter.

## Embodied reflexivity: Auto/body mapping

Prior to beginning the study, Helen engaged in what she calls *"auto/body mapping,"* creating her own body maps as an embodied approach to researcher reflexivity (Harrison, 2021) (see Figure 7.1). The body mapping method used by Solomon's (2002) and Gastaldo's (2012) research teams was adapted in two major ways. First, Helen had her body traced onto a large piece of paper while standing instead of lying down, which she experienced as contributing to a sense of agency during the process. Second, Eugene Gendlin's (1981) *"focusing"* method was used to scan her body for *"power points"* (Solomon, 2002, 27). In Gendlin's five-step method, the person:

1   clears a space to relax and turn attention inwardly to the body, asking what is being sensed in response to a question such as "what are my strengths as an educator?,"
2   selects one of the items sensed, paying attention to where it is felt in the body,
3   lets a word(s) or image/symbol come up from the felt sense, staying with the quality of the felt sense until the best fit is found via a word(s) or image/symbol,
4   goes back and forth between the felt sense and the word(s) or image/symbol to check how they resonate with each other,
5   asks what it is about this felt sense that makes it resonate with the word(s) or image/symbol chosen (1981, 50–51).

The process deeply informed Helen's insights about the method and provided an experiential foundation to work with. In addition, Helen gained insights into her assumptions, vulnerabilities and strengths as a learner and teacher. An additional

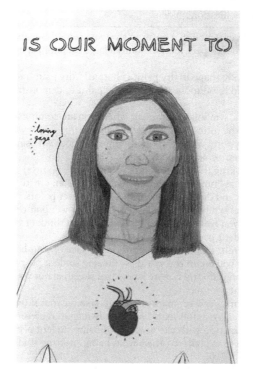

*Figure 7.1* Helen's Auto/Body Map – Educator Strengths: Loving Gaze and Heart

auto-body map as "researcher" nurtured further insights regarding her interactions with participants and the research team – a more detailed elaboration of this process is described elsewhere (Harrison, 2021).

## Body map facilitation guide

The body-mapping guidelines were adapted from the work of both Solomon (2002) and Gastaldo (2012) as a research method to guide questions and facilitate the body map process (see Table 7.3).

In step 5 (body scan), participants engaged in the process of "focusing" so that their "bodily felt sense" of powerful points in the body was evoked, rather than only their filtered cognitive thoughts. The focusing method led the participant to step 6, in which they drew their "power" symbols in the relevant places on the map.

## Body map data: Exemplars

Participants described differences between what insights arose in the face-to-face interview and the body mapping sessions. Several peer mentors shared impressions that this arts-based method evoked more connection among ideas, deeper reflection, and engagement of emotions than interviews alone.

*Table 7.3* Body map facilitation guide

| | |
|---|---|
| 1 | Trace your body in pencil in a position that says something about your experience as a "nursing student peer mentor" onto a large sheet of paper (may have help of partner). |
| 2 | Highlight the body shape in dry paint (Sharpie™ dry paint pens, water based) or markers and add hand/footprints in acrylic paint to demonstrate their presence in the world. |
| 3 | Choose and draw symbols to represent where you are coming from and what your dreams are for the future as a student nurse/nurse. |
| 4 | Paint in your support: Write the (nick)names of those who support you as a nursing student/peer mentor on the body map. |
| 5 | Body scan – marking the power points: Visualise the point(s) on your body that give you power as "nursing student peer mentor" then create personal symbols to represent them and draw them on or near the power points. |
| 6 | Create a personal symbol: Draw a symbol on the power points on the map that represent how you feel about yourself and how you think of yourself in the world as "nursing student peer mentor." |
| 7 | Draw a self-portrait: Draw a self-portrait on the face of your body tracing that represents how you are in the world as "nursing student peer mentor." |
| 8 | Creating a personal slogan: Create a personal slogan about your strengths as a "nursing student peer mentor." |
| 9 | Marks on the skin: Draw on marks that you have on your skin (physical) and under the skin (physical or emotional) on the body map to represent physical and emotional interaction with the world as "nursing student peer mentor." |
| 10 | Create a symbol to explain to others what being "nursing student peer mentor" means to you. |
| 11 | Public message: Message to the general public about becoming a "nursing student peer mentor." |
| 12 | Add more drawings, symbols or colours to the rest of the body map until you are satisfied that it (partially) represents you. |

Sources: Adapted from Gastaldo et al., (2012); Solomon (2002).

EXEMPLAR 1: Summer shared her perception that body mapping involved her emotions and increased clarity of her thinking:

> I think you asked something in the [face to face] interview about your body, think about what parts [and senses] might be involved. But for me, ... drawing it out made it easier for me to understand my feelings about it, rather than talking. I actually felt like I was able to think about it a little bit more clearly.

EXEMPLAR 2: Figure 7.2 offers an exemplar of a body map created during the study that is also used as an exemplar for the collaborative analysis process described later in the chapter.

Following Ellingson (2006), Helen also paid attention to intercorporeal bodily interactions during body-mapping sessions. The sessions were video recorded (for those consenting) and photos were taken to "show" bodily relations among participants, the researcher (Helen), and the body maps. Helen tried to remain

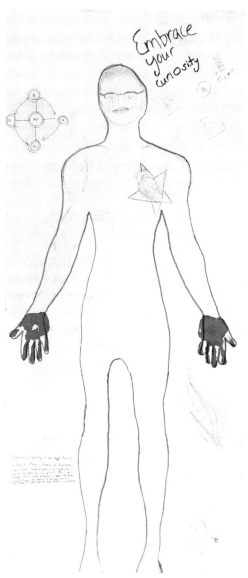

*Figure 7.2* Body Map of Participant Co-Researcher "James"

open to participants' corporeal needs. For example, partway through a 4-hour body-mapping session, participants stated that their bodies were achy from working on body maps, and an impromptu yoga session emerged, with one participant as the leader and other participants and Helen as yoga classmates. This spontaneous change in response to the bodies in attendance was an example of how attention to intercorporeality was employed in space and time.

## Embodied data analysis

The three philosophical insights on embodiment, intersubjectivity and intercorporeality also informed the design of the analysis plan.[5] The plan used an embodied approach to:

a  identify emergent themes from the interview data (Finlay, 2009; Wright-St. Clair, 2015),

b  engage Gendlin's (1962) idea of "felt sense" to discern meaning from the data, and

c  draw on embodied processes developed by Mallin (1996) to analyse the visual data.

Parts a) and b) above are outlined in the "Embodied Hermeneutic Analysis of Interview Data" section, and c) is outlined in "Embodied Hermeneutic Analysis of Body map Data" section below.

To honour participants' experiences and to collaborate within an intersubjective, dialogic space, we invited participants to join with the original research team in the data analysis processes. To participate in this way, students needed to have completed the nursing research course offered in the second year of their program. To satisfy ethical considerations, participants only engaged in analysis of their own data in collaboration with the primary researcher (Helen). Participants did not analyse other participants' interview transcripts or body maps, and, as per ethics approval, joining the research team in the analysis stages was entirely voluntary.

## Embodied hermeneutic analysis of interview data

Following Wright-St Clair's work (2015), we drew out stories that showed striking examples of the phenomena. In this process, we moved between parts of key stories and insights to the research transcripts in their entirety and back again as they illuminated and evoked the phenomena. We ensured that the parts and the whole were mutually reflective of one another, following Gadamer's (1975) and Heidegger's (1992) notions of a hermeneutic circle.

While transcripts were being prepared, Helen began initial data analysis using her memory of what participants had expressed during interviews. She incorporated attention to the "felt sense" (Gendlin, 1962) of the initial meanings being brought forth in the interview data – the embodied interpretation achieved through Gendlin's "focusing" tends to contain more action words and more bodily feeling descriptors than may come to mind through cognitive thinking alone. Helen interwove Mallin's (1996) "cognitive-linguistic" and "motor-practical" styles of interpretation by thinking about interviews while walking briskly on a treadmill and entering ideas that came to mind into her cell phone.

When the transcriptions were available, Helen read one transcript, then "slept on it" and developed a hand-drawn mind map in the morning. This was an example of "dwelling while sleeping" or "embodied thinking" during sleep. In her dissertation, Elizaveta Solomonova (2017) argued that *"dreaming is an embodied process of sense-making in the dream world"* (iii). Although Helen did not have dreams that related specifically to the transcripts, it was Helen's impression that some processing of the participants' words occurred during sleep.

Early in the analysis, Helen and Elizabeth Anne met to start the analysis of one transcript together and to sketch out initial themes identified in the data. Mind maps were developed for interview data of several participants, and an intersubjective analysis was subsequently carried out. Helen met with participants who accepted the invitation to analyse data and asked them to "mind map" themes identified in their own interview transcripts. In these face-to-face meetings, manuscripts were read by researcher and participant co-researcher in the same space and time. Mind maps were compared, and areas of convergence and divergence noted. Four or five themes were drawn out of each mind map and themes were colour coded. Each person read the transcript a second time, highlighting specific passages that illuminated rich examples of the themes. If a passage was especially salient or powerful, a star was written beside it in the margin (see Figure 7.3).

Not all participants volunteered to analyse data. In these cases, faculty team members were involved so that more than one person participated in the analysis of each transcript. Elizabeth Anne engaged in this process for several transcripts to cross-check for consistency and trustworthiness in the process. Subsequently, using themes from all mind maps, we used the program Quirkos™ (https://www.quirkos.com/) to begin organising the subthemes into groups. Helen paid attention to her "gut sense" of themes that were being identified in the transcripts as she read each one in its entirety and then read the parts of them that had been colour coded into initial tentative themes in Quirkos™.

In moving back and forth between the parts and whole of each transcript, and between the varying ways that aspects of our bodies understood and made meaning of the participants' words, we experienced what could be described as an *embodied* hermeneutic. According to Merleau-Ponty, the body brings forth understanding of situations from a multitude of sensations and perceptions through its own unity. He writes:

> It is not me who touches, but rather my body. When I touch I do not conceive of a multiplicity … I can only effectively touch if the phenomenon encounters an echo in me … The unity and the identity of the tactile phenomenon are not produced through a synthesis of recognition in the concept, they are established upon the unity and the identity of the body as a synergetic whole. (2012, 330)

Once this analysis process was completed for each transcript, an analysis of predominant themes across transcripts for peer mentors was undertaken. This involved a number of meetings and ongoing iterative dialogues between research team members and mind mapping of consolidated thematic representations of a) teaching, b) learning and c) relationships of peer mentorship.

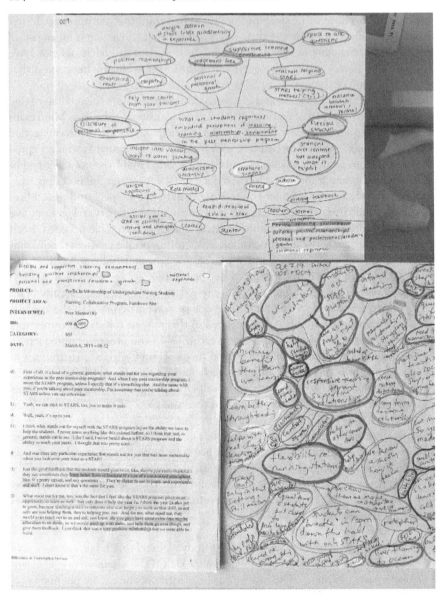

*Figure 7.3* Photograph of Colour-Coded[6] Mind Map Themes by Helen & Participant
Co-Researcher Sophie

## Embodied hermeneutic analysis of body map data

Ideas from scholars who draw on Merleau-Ponty's work – particularly those of
Mallin[7] – were incorporated into the body map data analysis plan. Mallin used an
embodied phenomenological approach to interpret both art and life situations; he
was especially interested in feminine/non-Eurocentric ways of seeing the world.

He argued that "*thinking based on 'lines,' or more bodily dimensions of existence …*
*has at least as much importance as [thinking] based on 'word'*" (1996, 239). Mallin
developed a "de-lineative" hermeneutics, which he used to analyse works of art in
an embodied manner.

When Mallin interpreted artworks, he included meanings gained from his "felt
bodily sense" of the work, along with detailed descriptions of the nature and
directions of lines in the art (1996, 16). We used a similar process to analyse body
maps; researchers assumed the pose depicted in the body map and focused on the
"felt sense" evoked. The directions of the lines of the body outline itself and other
elements on the maps were described and interpreted.

Mallin describes his "body hermeneutic method" based on five "regions"
of the body to interpret artwork or life situations: (1) cognitive-linguistic, 2)
emotional-social, (3) perceptual, (4) motor-practical and 5) visceral (2009,
24–25). Paying attention to how different aspects of one's body interprets
phenomena resonated with the aims of our study. Although these "regions"
may sound somewhat reductionist, conceptualising them instead as different "manners" or "styles" of coming to understand the phenomenon provided a useful way to approach analysis of the body maps. Mallin suggested
that directing attention to the "regions" may more wilfully invite bodily
meaning-making processes.

Considering these affordances, we incorporated Mallin's body hermeneutic
into our guide for analysing body maps and propose that it offers an original
approach to embodied data analysis methods (see Table 7.4).

*Table 7.4* Body map data analysis guide

---

1  What meanings and lived experiences are revealed about peer mentorship through
   the images, symbols, drawings and stories that were developed during creation of this
   body map?
   Focus on several different (but overlapping) manners of meaning-making:
   • cognitive-linguistic
   • emotional-social
   • perceptual
   • motor-practical (psychomotor)
   • visceral ("gut feeling")
2  What does this body map suggest to you about:
   • teaching
   • learning
   • relationships
   • the environment of peer mentorship?
3  What other questions could this body map answer?
4  What does the composition of the various elements inside and outside of the body on
   the map suggest about the experience of peer mentorship? Speak to your responses to
   the colour choices of the map's creator, that is, how do the colours shape your
   perceptions of the body map?
5  What do you experience bodily as you assume the pose of the person depicted in the
   body map?

---

Source: Informed by Works of Samuel Mallin.

During the body-mapping sessions, each participant described their reasons for choosing various symbols, colours and drawings, and these in-the-moment inter-pretations were given primary importance in the analysis. As the first "audience" of the maps, the researchers observed and recorded their own responses to the maps. These observations were shared with participants during the collaborative analysis process. Through iterative dialogue, interpretations of researchers and participants were included in the findings. All research team members were key in working towards a coherent interpretation and analysis of the visual and tex-tual data set. Examples of our collaborative interpretations are described next.

## Embodied data analysis with participant co-researchers

Given varying styles of analysing visual data, we maintained a flexible approach to data analysis with participant co-researchers. Prior to meeting with Helen, the following guidelines were emailed to the participants:

> As you look at your body map, try to imagine you are seeing it for the first time when you think about answering the questions. If you don't want to do the parts of question 1 separately, you don't have to. Just, however you want, describe what you see holistically. You can type your answers into the Word document or jot them down on a separate piece of paper to refer to during our meeting. Please let me know if you have questions.

When participants met with Helen, they shared their interpretations first, fol-lowed by our interpretations. Participants were then asked about resonance or disparity of interpretation.

Here are two illustrative quotes excerpted from a single body map analysis Zoom meeting:

PARTICIPANT/CO-RESEARCHER JAMES: Cognitively, my message to the public shows a rational analysis of mentorship regarding knowledge transmission, facilitating holism, and passing on wisdom. The green outline [of the body] shows consideration of nursing as a positive experience. Emotional-socially, the slogan [embrace your curiosity] and open hands show openness to inter-actions with others making it a nurturing setting. The warmth of the smile represents shared kindness to facilitate growth. The body map suggests that the experience is positive and a reciprocal mutually beneficial relationship between teacher and learning ... and the bright flame beside the body implies the passion that is involved with peer mentorship in nursing. Perceptually, symbols of my peers, knowledge, professors, and the mentees, represents perception of interactions of the lab being a space of wholeness/influence received and influence given, of mutual relations. The question mark symbol shows perceiving nursing as being a little bit mysterious (can't quite define it) and perceiving the strength built through these interactions as a peer mentor. Motor-practically, the hands are red, implying sharing knowledge of nursing through hands on assessments. Viscerally, the drawing of the heart embodies physiological sense, muscles as strength, flame being a physical sense of warmth. When I assume this pose, I feel a sense of power and pride from standing in this position, and a sense of grounding to the earth, as providing a certain level of stability.

RESEARCHER HELEN: Cognitively, I notice the peer mentor in the body map giving a direct gaze, suggesting eye contact and engagement with the viewer. Emotional-socially, the open posture and smile and grounded feet give me a sense of being able to trust the peer mentor. Perceptually, I notice that vision is depicted as prominent among the senses. The sketches of the muscles reveal a possible role of kinesthesia/proprioception in the peer mentorship process, perhaps potential movements in response to mentees. The prominence of the hands suggests the sense of touch being important in the peer mentorship process. Motor-practically, the prominence of the muscles and hands speak to a dynamic sense of potential motion at any time and in any direction, perhaps depending on what the mentee needs. The hands appear ready to show or gesture to assist learning or growth. Viscerally, my gut sense is that I can trust this person. The hands appear strong and open to helping. The fire beside the mentor does intimidate me somewhat as I am an introvert and I fear having to match the level of passion of the peer mentor. When I am in this pose, I feel strong but open and inviting connection. Grounded.

When James was presented with Helen's interpretation of his body map, he indicated that all aspects resonated with him. He particularly liked the observations that he looked trustworthy and that his depiction of his muscles seemed to evoke a proprioceptive awareness of how his muscles needed to move in response to his mentees. On occasion, a participant-coresearcher did not sense a resonance with the way a researcher interpreted an aspect of their body maps. In these cases, the interpretation of the participant was prioritised. For example, one participant had drawn pink wavy lines inside the lungs on her body map. While Helen sensed movement, and the possibility of "breathing with" mentees, the participant stated that movement was not her intended meaning – she was only trying to colour in the lungs quickly.

## Sharing findings with participants

Honouring a collaborative approach, the themes identified in the analysis of one data set were sent to participants by email, including the participants who declined to join the analysis team. Six of the seven themes were given a "phenomenological nod"[8] by the peer mentors. One participant and one faculty research team member did not resonate with the theme named "offering generous acceptance" – both preferred the theme name "offering trustworthy support." In keeping with our intersubjective hermeneutic approach, we accepted this plurality in interpretation in meaning. We decided on themes which generated greater consensus while also including discussion about the different interpretations in the manuscript; we Included the theme name that resonated with most participants *plus* a section on distinct interpretations in the resulting manuscript (Harrison et al., 2021).

## Affordances, joys and challenges

There were many affordances of using an embodied hermeneutic phenomenological approach. We were able to commit to valuing embodiment, intersubjectivity and intercorporeality throughout the research process, providing a rich, embodied perspective. Inviting participants to join the study as co-researchers served to decrease a sense of hierarchy. In some ways, while studying peer mentorship among nursing students, Helen was acting as a "qualitative research mentor" to the participant-researchers while also being mentored, herself, by more experienced members of the research team *and* by the participants. We were able to maintain a multidimensional perspective during all phases of the research. There were natural differences in style and approaches to an analysis by different team members – however, many commonalities of themes and interpretations were identified by the multiple people engaged in the analysis. Since their experience was being investigated, we prioritised the participants' interpretations.

Joys included "dwelling" in the data and developing collegial "peer" relationships with participants (especially those engaging in analyses). We experienced joy when participants replied by email confirming their interest to engage in data analysis when they shared stories regarding their body maps or reflected on the resonance of themes identified in the data. Also, participants shared their excitement about the research, which in turn nurtured research capacity in undergraduate students. The embodied nature of the investigation generated great richness of the data, which is different in quality from any other known research in the area of student peer mentorship. This addressed the call for more embodied and relational research in higher education and professional education settings (Perry and Medina, 2011).

Challenges included the intense study and time required to become fluent with Merleau-Ponty's work and to distil elements of his work into the practice of phenomenology. The study generated voluminous data from interviews, body maps, and videos of body-mapping sessions. With over 70 hours of recorded data, the research team needed to make difficult decisions about how to distribute the data, stories and images for representation in different reports of the findings. Given the busy schedules of faculty and students, challenges with scheduling analysis meetings arose. In addition, we were cautious not to "over-interpret" the visual data or make "leading" suggestions in analysis with participants.

One pitfall that arose was the arrival of the COVID-19 pandemic, which led to the need for online meetings for collaborative body map analysis. This decreased our ability to be in the same place and time as participants, but ironically increased people's availability to meet; we adapted by using photographs of the body maps to send to participants and holding meetings via Zoom to engage in dialogue about analyses of the maps.

# Conclusion

Our aim in this chapter has been to conceptualise and articulate an embodied hermeneutic phenomenological methodology and to show how such a design was fruitfully employed in research into peer mentorship. We hope the time invested in working through Merleau-Ponty's thought and how it could be applied in a practical way might be an important contribution to the conversation among qualitative researchers. In particular, we propose that the theoretical work of Merleau-Ponty, Gendlin and Mallin can advance a deeper level of engagement with embodied perceptions in hermeneutic phenomenological research.

# Notes

1. Approval for the research on student peer mentorship was obtained from the research ethics board of the educational institutions. Ten participants were recruited, with an age range of 19–26 years (average 21.1 years), seven identifying as male, two identifying as female and one declining to identify gender.
2. Gestalt being a German term that roughly translates to "how something is put together" – Britannica online dictionary.
3. Interlocutors: Persons who take part in a dialogue or conversation.
4. Standardised patients are actors hired to role play a client with a particular health challenge to enable students of health professions to practice clinical skills in a safe environment.
5. Available from the authors on request Email: hfharris@uwo.ca
6. The map is not reproduced here in its original colour and appears in greyscale. If you wish to see the maps in colour, contact the authors directly (as per note 5).
7. This included his unpublished work The Body on My Mind: Body Hermeneutics (Mallin 2009).
8. Phenomenological nod in this context means that "a good phenomenological description is something that we can nod to, recognizing as an experience that we have had or could have had …. a good phenomenological description is collected by lived experience and recollects lived experience" (van Manen, 1990, 27).

# References

Andersen, T. and Watkins, K. (2018). The Value of Peer Mentorship as an Educational Strategy. Nursing. Journal of Nursing Education 57(4): 217–224.

Cuffari, E. and Streeck, J. (2017). Taking the World by Hand: How (Some) Gestures Mean. In: Meyer, C., Streeck, J. and Jordan, J. S. (eds), Intercorporeality: Emerging Socialities in Interaction. Oxford University Press, Oxford.

Davey, N. (1999). The Hermeneutics of Seeing. In: Heywood, I. and Sandywell, B. (eds) Interpreting Visual Culture: Explorations in the Hermeneutics of the Visual (pp. 3–29). Routledge, London.

de Jager, A., Tewson, A., Ludlow, B., and Boydell, K. (2016). Embodied Ways of Storying the Self: A Systematic Review of Body-Mapping. Forum: Qualitative Social Research 17(2): 1–31.

Dowling, M. (2007). From Husserl to van Manen: A Review of Different Phenomenological Approaches. International Journal of Nursing Studies 44: 131–142.

Ellingson, L. (2006). Embodied Knowledge: Writing Researchers' Bodies into Qualitative Health Research. Qualitative Health Research 16(2): 298–310.

Finlay, L. (2009). Exploring lived experience: Principles and practice of phenomenological research. International Journal of Therapy and Rehabilitation 16(9), pp. 474–481.

Gadamer, H.-G. (1975). Truth and Method. Continuum, New York, NY. (Original work published 1960.)

Gastaldo, D., Magalhaes, L., Carrasco, C., and Davy, C. (2012). Body-Map Storytelling as Research: Methodological Considerations for Telling the Stories of Undocumented Workers through Body Mapping. Retrieved online 1 May 2019: https://migration health.ca/sites/default/files/Body-map_storytelling_as_reseach_LQ.pdf

Gendlin, E. T. (1962). Experiencing and the Creation of Meaning. Free Press, Glencoe, NY.

Gendlin, E. T. (1981). Focusing. Bantam Books, New York.

Gooding, A. (1968). SomaPsyche. Unpublished manuscript.

Green, W. (2015) Thinking Bodies: Practice Theory, Deleuze, and Professional Education. In: Green, B. and Hopwood, N. (eds) The Body in Professional Practice, Learning and Education. Professional and Practice-Based Learning, vol. 11. Springer, Cham. https://doi.org/10.1007/978-3-319-00140-1_15

Guenther, L. (2019). Critical Phenomenology. In: Weiss, G., et al. (eds) 50 Concepts for a Critical Phenomenology. Northwestern University Press, Evanston, IL.

Guillemin, M. and Drew, S. (2010). Questions of Process in Participant-Generated Visual Methodologies. Visual Studies 25(2): 175–188.

Harrison, H. F. (2021). Body Mapping to Facilitate Embodied Reflection in Professional Education Programs. In: Loftus, S. and Kinsella, E. A. (eds) Embodiment and Professional Education: Body, Practice, Pedagogy. Springer Nature. https://doi.org/10.1007/978-981-16-4827-4_8

Harrison, H. F., Kinsella, E., and DeLuca, S. (2019) Locating the Lived Body in Client–Nurse Interactions: Embodiment, Intersubjectivity and Intercorporeality. Nursing Philosophy 20(2). https://doi.org/10.1111/nup.12241

Harrison, H. F., Kinsella, E., DeLuca, S., and Loftus, S. (2021). "We Know What They're Struggling with": Student Peer Mentors' Embodied Perceptions of Teaching in a Health Professional Education Mentorship Program. https://doi.org/10.1007/s10459-021-10072-9

Heidegger, M. (1992). The Metaphysical Foundations of Logic. Translated by M. Heim. Bloomington and Indianapolis: Indiana University Press.

Kinsella, E. A. (2006) Hermeneutics and Critical Hermeneutics: Exploring Possibilities within the Art of Interpretation. Forum Qualitative Sozial forschung/Forum: Qualitative Social Research [Online Journal], May, 7(3), Art. 19. Available at: http://www.qualitative-research.net/fqs-texte/3-06/06-3-19-e.htm

Kinsella, E. A. (2009). Professional Knowledge and the Epistemology of Reflective Practice. Nursing Philosophy 11(1): 3–14.

Kinsella, E. A. (2012). Practitioner Reflection and Judgement as Phronesis: A Continuum of Reflection and Considerations for Phronetic Judgement. In: Kinsella, E. A. and Pitman, A. (eds) Phronesis as Professional Knowledge: Practical Wisdom in the Professions. Sense Publishing, Rotterdam.

Kinsella E. A. and Bidinosti, S. (2015). "I Now Have a Visual Image in My Mind and It Is Something I Will Never Forget": An Analysis of an Arts-Informed Approach to Health Professions Ethics Education. Advances in Health Sciences Education 21: 303–322. DOI 10.1007/s10459-015-9628-7

Lakoff, G. and Johnson, M., 2008. Metaphors We Live By. Chicago: University of Chicago Press.

Mallin, S. (1996). Art, Line Thought. Kluwer Academic Publishers, Boston.

Mallin, S. (2009). The Body on My Mind: Body Hermeneutics. Unpublished book, York University.

McCorquodale, L. and DeLuca, S. (2020). You Want Me to Draw What? Body Mapping in Qualitative Research as Canadian Socio-Political Commentary. Forum, Qualitative Social Research 21(2). https://doi.org/10.17169/fqs-21.2.3242

McKenna, L. and Williams, B. (2017). The Hidden Curriculum in Near-Peer Learning: An Exploratory Qualitative Study. Nurse Education Today 50: 77–81.

Merleau-Ponty, M. (1962, 2012). Phenomenology of Perception. Routledge, New York, NY. (Original work published 1945).

Merleau-Ponty, M. (1964). Signs. Northwestern University Press, Evanston, IL.

Orchard, T. (2017). Remembering the Body: Ethical Issues in Body Mapping Research. Springer, New York.

Perry, M. and Medina, C. (2011). Embodiment and Performance in Pedagogy Research: Investigating the Possibility of the Body in Curriculum Experience. Journal of Curriculum Theorizing 27(3): 62–75.

Ramm, D., Thomson, A., and Jackson, A. (2015). Learning Clinical Skills in the Simulation Suite: The Lived Experiences of Student Nurses Involved in Peer Teaching and Peer Assessment. Nurse Education Today 35: 823–827.

Solomon, J. (2002). Living with X: A Body-Mapping Journey in Time of HIV and AIDS. Facilitator's Guide. Psychosocial Wellbeing Series. REPSSI, Johannesburg, South Africa.

Solomonova, E. (2017). The Embodied Mind in Sleep and Dreaming: A Theoretical Framework and an Empirical Study of Sleep, Dreams and Memory in Meditators and Controls, Dissertation, University of Montreal.

Wright-St. Clair, V. A. (2015). Doing (Interpretive) Phenomenology. In: Stanley, M. and Nayar, S. (eds) Qualitative Research Methodologies for Occupational Science and Therapy. Routledge, London.

van Manen, M. (1990). Researching Lived Experience: Human Science for an Action Sensitive Pedagogy. State University of New York Press, Albany, NY.

# 8 Dwelling in the fourfold

## My way of being-in-the-world of Heidegger

*Margot Solomon*

## Abstract

Hermeneutic phenomenology, as elucidated by Martin Heidegger, is used both as a methodology to guide method and as a springboard to thinking about how the teacher learns as she teaches. The focus was on "my" teaching, drawing from my journals and nineteen self-focused interviews with colleagues and ex-students. The hermeneutics-of-self challenges the researcher to be both inside and outside the research recognising, in amongst the familiar, what has been hidden and/or taken-for-granted.

The notions that Heidegger uses illustrate through a philosophical lens what it is to be human. The *fourfold* and *dwelling* are two of these notions and underpin the structure of my data analysis. The fourfold is an integral part of any *thing*. Together the four elements of the fourfold (sky, earth, mortals and divinities) are present in a moment when the object becomes a *thing*. Heidegger writes of dwelling as belonging within the fourfold, where parts gather into the whole. The fourfold offers a structure that provides a primordial relatedness to the phenomena being studied. I used dwelling in the fourfold as a structure for the themes that emerge in my thesis, drawing on the philosophy of Heidegger.

## Introduction

I had been attending a Heidegger monthly seminar at the university for many years, so his notions were both familiar and engaging. The philosophical assumptions resonated with my psychoanalytic psychotherapy theoretical understanding. Both are interpretive, acknowledge the context, and are interested in what is hidden and taken for granted. Because my quest was to find meaning within the "how" of my own teaching, I reframed the usual manner of interpreting the text of others to engage in a hermeneutics-of-self. I did this by a combination of being interviewed by colleagues that knew my teaching to pull forth my own stories of being a teacher and by interviewing ex-students. Colleagues asked about my experience of teaching, while I invited ex-students to tell stories about being in my classes. It was an opportunity to reflect on how I practiced teaching psychotherapy and to give back my learning to future teachers. Kenneth Fleck, Liz Smythe and John Hitchens argue that the hermeneutics-of-self offers an opportunity for the researcher to "*dwell with what is closest which is often the hardest to see*" (Fleck et al., 2011, 27). Through this highly personal revelation comes a depth that is seldom revealed.

DOI: 10.4324/9781003081661-8

While all hermeneutic phenomenological research requires researchers to consider their own fore-structure, the hermeneutics-of-self involves self-observation, which is defined as *"the capacity to observe the self and its relations to others in the present moment"* (Falkenstrom, 2007, 552). Fleck et al. (2011) is the first piece of research that I have been able to find that directly uses the hermeneutics-of-self as a method supported by the philosophy of Heidegger and Gadamer. As a psychotherapist, I am familiar with the method of self-observation (Falkenstrom, 2007), reverie and reflection (Solomon, 2014; 2017). All these terms are used to describe at different levels the capacity to notice one's own experience and make meaning of it. The hermeneutics-of-self uses the researcher to access experiences that are difficult to bring-into-view. It is the researcher's experience of the phenomenon; in this case, teaching and learning. At the centre of my findings is the notion of "learning and teaching as relating," which means that the relationship between teacher and students is intrinsic to effective teaching and learning. In this chapter, I will begin by defining the Heideggerian notions I used including, dwelling, thing and fourfold. Then I will describe and illustrate my process of analysis and interpretation, followed by two examples from the data in my doctorate.

## Dwelling

When thinking about the journey I undertook to use Heidegger's thinking in my thesis, it involved pathways of reading Heidegger, keeping a journal alongside studying the interviews, and belonging to a Heidegger reading group – it is amazing how much more sense can be made when a group of people convene together to think about a piece of Heideggerian text. Dwelling was the most important activity. Dwelling on all of the above, and, dwelling as occurring in a familiar and ordinary way, just as Heidegger (1998, 270) describes through the story of Heraclitus, the thinker who said, *"For here too the Gods are present"* while engaging in standing by the fire warming himself.

Dwelling is the core activity that took me into the realm of Heidegger's ideas. Heidegger (2001) pointed towards "building out of dwelling" and thinking as the way that the nature of dwelling can be experienced. Heidegger differentiates between essential dwelling, present in us all and part of what makes us human, being-at-home, safe and taking care; and an *"existential dwelling which consists in understanding one's essential dwelling and living in the light of that understanding"* (Young, 2002, 74). Dwelling is about finding peace in one's existence, accepting the thrownness (our lack of control over where and when our existence begins, endures and ends) of existence as it shows up, going with the flow while grappling with the human tendency to control the world rather than to "spare" it (take care of or facilitate its natural unfolding).

One of the limits working with the English translation of Heidegger's works is that I am distanced from Heidegger's thinking. Most importantly, he explored the meanings derived from the roots of words in German. My experience is that something is always lost in translation and over time. I also discovered that different translations use different English words. Thus, I found it useful to explore the etymology of words. Words have a history, and thus the older meanings are embedded in newer understandings. Etymology helps to see what is hidden and more possibilities in the meaning of what is being said. An example is trying to unpack the way Heidegger links dwell (*wohnen*) with build (*bauen*). It is clearer in German than English. The English word dwell cited in Etymonline.com links to old English "to lead into error" to middle English "to procrastinate" and eventually "to linger, remain, stay." These words do not connect to my understanding of building. However, when I looked at the etymological story of build, the link back to dwell was found; Proto-Germanic *buthla – from PIE *bhu- "to dwell," from root*bheue- "to be, exist, grow." Building could be related to "a dwelling," where dwelling is a noun. When both are used as verbs, they can relate to creating a safe space where one's essential being can grow. Then, in the reading group, I discovered that another text by Heidegger (1993) referred directly to the same etymological connections. Heidegger shows us his way of thinking, he constantly asks questions that deepen the possible meaning of the ideas he is discussing. There is an openness in his questioning, a curiosity about the derivation of the meanings of the words he is using, as the example above illustrates. This openness is a reflection of his approach to philosophy as ontological rather than ontic.[1]

Existential dwelling is about finding meaning and, in so doing, touching the primordial and living in that space. Dwelling is accepting a *thing* the way it is, being present to it and at the same time being open to thinking about it from many perspectives. This is the way to work with the transcripts from interviews and with reading Heidegger. There is an ineffable process that goes on that does not happen in the conscious mind. Heidegger said, "... *human being [Dasein] consists in dwelling and, indeed dwelling in the sense of the stay of mortals on the earth ... under the sky ... remaining before the divinities... and includes a belonging to men's being with one another*" (Heidegger, 1993, 351). Dwelling is the guardian of the fourfold (Heidegger, 2001, 149). With that in mind, I will now describe the fourfold.

## The fourfold

The fourfold has been cited as Heidegger's least understood concept (Harman, 2007; Mitchell, 2015). The fourfold is a structure which describes the world. They cannot be separated because all elements are a mirror-play of each other, they all reflect each other back to each other. Heidegger describes it thus:

> Each of the four in its way mirrors the essence of the remaining others again. Each is thus reflected in its way back into what is its own within the single fold of the four. This mirroring is no presentation of an image. Lighting up each of the four, this mirroring appropriates the essence of each to the others in a simple bringing into ownership.
>
> (Heidegger, 2012, 17)

Further, the fourfold are structures that herald the difference between an object and a *thing*[2]; it specifies and gives depth and meaning to the *thing*. The existence of this or that *thing* is determined by the mirror-play of the fourfold. A central tenet of the fourfold is that while each of its four aspects is being thought of, the other three are already in our minds "by the simple oneness of the four" (Heidegger, 2001). Thus, the earth is the bearer, the ground that brings forth. As the earth needs a medium through which it can appear, this is the sky. The sky is the movement of the planets and stars, the changing of the seasons, the turning of day and night, as well as the weather. It is that which we can see but cannot influence. The divinities are the messengers of the Godhead (Heidegger, 2001, 147–8). Julian Young (2002) describes the divinities as *"the (appropriated or unappropriated) guidance of a particular ethical heritage"* (98). I consider the divinities to be the receiving of understanding from the deeper knowing we all carry inside; it is the culture we live in that touches the collective unconscious of humanity and brings forth a primordial type of knowing. Mitchell succinctly says, "the divinities name the meaning of a *thing*" (Mitchell, 2015, 210). Our unconscious processes sit here with our gods and the mystery that remains hidden. Mortals are human beings, and our consciousness of our own mortality is what distinguishes us as human, as mortal. It is through dwelling that mortals enter the fourfold (Heidegger, 2001).

## The thing

The fourfold is always relating to the *thing*. Every-*thing* in the world is in a relationship with every-*thing* else. Figure 8.1 summarises the fourfold as intrinsically connected to the thing. The elements on the outside of the circle represent what will become the fourfold in my thesis. As Mitchell says, *"there is nothing*

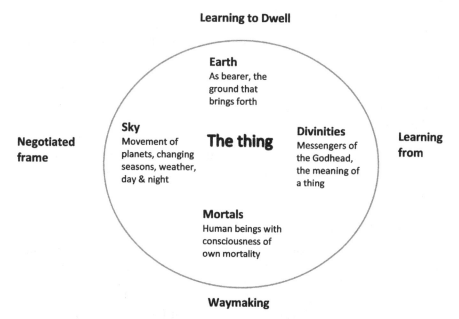

*Figure 8.1* The Thing and the Fourfold

*that does not exist in this relational way;"* it is *"the hospitality of things"* (Mitchell, 2015, 5). Gathering of the fourfold is what makes it a *thing* rather than an object. Heidegger discusses the origin of the word *thing* as meaning *"a gathering, ... to deliberate on a matter under discussion"* (Heidegger, 2001, 172). It is human engagement that makes the transition from object to *thing.* Heidegger's example of the jug is a case in point. The fourfold could be represented as follows: the earth is the context/the situation in which the jug will be used. Perhaps I am expecting a visitor to my home. The jug sits as an object in my kitchen. Sky is the thrown aspects out of my control. When my visitor arrives, I will offer her a drink. I do not know what she might like. Unexpectedly my visitor brings flowers. I am the mortal in my situated connectedness who reaches for the jug, a perfect holder of the flowers. In the background are the divinities, represented in this instance by the custom my visitor has to bring gifts when visiting. My custom is to offer a drink to any visitor. The jug has become a thing. It has been used. The using of the jug is the *as-ness,* when it becomes a particular jug used in a particular way. The jug *as* a holder of milk, for example, to offer to guests when they come for a cup of tea. The jug is used to hold something in particular. That is how the jug (*thing*) presences. The jug could be used to hold flowers. The thingness of the jug then changes. Heidegger said, the *thing* things (Heidegger, 2001, 172). How does the *thing* presence, how does the *thing* at the centre of my study show itself? Teaching and learning are like the jug, not as "object" but as a jug-in-play, showing itself afresh every day. The purpose of the teaching and learning, the *asness,* that which particularises my teaching and learning is "relating."

Heidegger said about the jug, *"the vessel's thingness does not lie at all in the material of which it consists, but in the void that holds"* (Heidegger, 2001, 167). The void that holds is the invisible, unconsidered part of the jug and yet also the essential component of the jug without which it could never be a jug. It is only through the gathering of the fourfold that the essence of the thing is revealed. The metaphor of the void in the jug – as that which is the centre of the use the jug is put to – exercised my mind. What was the equivalent in my thesis? In a way, the void in the jug is the real phenomenon, something always open to possibility. The jug is necessary to frame the void. Ah ha!, so in my thesis, learning is like that; teaching is the action (void) I am engaged in shaped by everything that makes it possible (the fourfold). Learning is implied but cannot be taken for granted. How do we know learning is happening? How does my teaching encounter invite learning?

## Overview of results

Once I had understood something of what Heidegger meant by the fourfold, I was able to see the structure of my findings. It did not happen all of a sudden. Rather it emerged like the dawning of a new day, new but connected to previous days. The *thing* revealed itself as teaching and learning as relating: the *Negotiated Frame*[3] (sky), *Learning to Dwell* (earth), *Way-making* (mortals) and *Learning From* (divinities). I used the sky to represent the *negotiated frame* as the sky holds many contexts that can be hospitable and inhospitable but also are essentially out of my control. The *negotiated frame* includes the "releasement towards things," "dynamic administration," "culture and difference" and "asymmetrical mutuality." The sky encloses and gives form to the earth. Earth is *learning to dwell*, as it holds the ground that makes it possible for me as a teacher to bring forth learning as I teach. *Learning to dwell* includes the themes of "grounding" myself, "being open," "letting the mind be a thoroughfare" and "creating space." Mortals represent the third element of *way-making*. Each student brings herself to the teaching and learning moments in her own way. She brings her past and her present and takes herself off into the future with the outpouring of the whole teaching-and-learning-as-relating experience. *Way-making* points the way; it outlines the journey my students and I go through in a teaching year. From "offering" to "holding," from "dissonance" to "creating a space for dialogue" and finally, "learning to think." The divinities are "*learning from*," because there are so many possible ways of understanding, of being-with what can never be known. The messages we receive in dreams and reveries lead us to our own meaning. Our unconscious processes sit here with our gods and the mystery that remains hidden. "*Learning from*" tracks the deeper processing of experience. It is "dreaming and reverie," "reflection," brought together into "intersubjective space" and "learning from experience."

Figure 8.2 summarises the data as a series of progressions. However, what is missed in this one-dimensional image is the constant presence of all the four elements with each other. The overlapping circles in the middle of Figure 8.2 are an attempt to show the fourfold as "*the simple onefold of earth and sky, of divinities and mortals*" (Heidegger, 2001, 155). The phenomenon is the thing at the centre of the study, in this case: Teaching and learning as relating.

## My process

Process is a word often used, but perhaps what is being communicated is not always understood. Process just goes where it goes, it has its own volition. That is something essential about the process. We are not in control. I am using the word process to mean a series of events or experiences that have coherence, that are linked together. Freud, when discussing the impact of the analyst's interventions, said the following:

> He (the analyst) sets in motion a process, that of the resolving of existing repressions. He can supervise this process, further it, removes obstacles in its way, and he can undoubtedly vitiate much of it. But on the whole, once begun, it goes its own way and does not allow either the direction it takes or the order in which it picks up its points to be prescribed for it.
>
> (Freud, 1913, 130)

Freud is talking about the process of healing in therapy. It is clear from this extract that the process has a goal (resolving existing repressions). My goal was

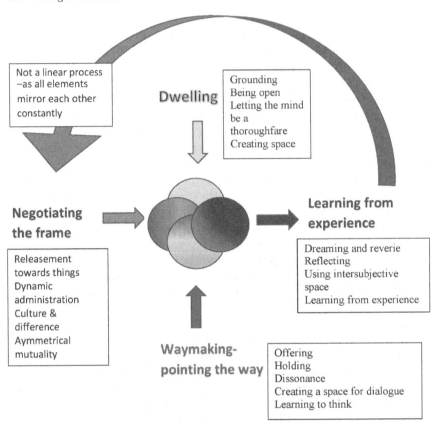

*Figure 8.2* The Phenomenon, Teaching and Learning as Relating

to explore how I learn as I teach using hermeneutic phenomenology. The Online Etymological Dictionary defines process as "fact of being carried on" (as in *process*), from Old French *process* "a journey; continuation, development; legal trial" (13c.) and directly from Latin *processus* "a going forward, advance, progress," from past participle stem of *procedere* "go forward." There is something about a process that can be recognised as a "continuous series of actions meant to accomplish some result" (https://www.etymonline.com/), and yet a process is unlikely to be seen clearly while in the middle of it, as it "goes its own way." It may be known after the event or experience is complete. When I look back at my journals, there were many moments where nothing at all was clear. All that I was aware of was that I would continue on the journey.

Heidegger used the idea of the forest path. I was on the path, unable to see the direction – there were too many trees. Looking back, I think the trees were all the little stories and emerging themes that could not quite fit together and yet were never really separate. When I look back over my method chapter, there is the dwelling that includes a long period of confusion and chaos, followed by some anxious trying to force the data into some kind of order, then having to let go, surrender to the process and continue on the forest path, not knowing where it was going. In common usage is the phrase "trust the process." For me, this originated in my gestalt therapy training in the 1980s. It is implicit for the therapist to trust the process (Brownell, 2016, 416). Likewise, my supervisors (who are of a similar age to me) often used the phrase in supervision when I got lost or tried to create order in my data before it naturally arose through the process.

Forcing the data was exemplified by my attempts at creating a clear structure through pinning down the chapter headings. These attempts lacked coherence. They reflected what I was holding on to, what I thought mattered. They reflected my anxiety about not knowing what was ahead, being lost on the forest path. These attempts at chapter headings are interspersed with records of dreams and my interpretations, reflection on teaching sessions, the day to day thoughts that relate to my thesis including connections to novels and films, thoughts as I listen to audio recordings of interviews, notes from Heidegger and other texts I was reading. All of this is gathering; a necessary antecedent to finding my way. I focused on the chapter headings whenever I felt lost or became anxious about deadlines.

So began a month of back and forth between trying to make sense of the fourfold and writing, the hermeneutic circle at work, allowing the themes that I had uncovered to begin to coalesce into bigger chunks of meaning. There were key questions my supervisor (our Heideggerian scholar) asked of the reading group. "What are you cherishing in your study? What is it in your study that is ripening?" I wrote them down and pondered them after the sessions. Below is the quote from Heidegger that inspired my supervisor's questions.

> To be a human being means to be on this earth as a mortal. It means to dwell. The old word *bauen*, which says that man *is* insofar as he *dwells*, this word *bauen* also means at the same time to cherish and to protect, to preserve and care for, specifically to toil the soil, to cultivate the vine. Such building only takes care – it tends the growth that ripens into its fruit of its own accord. Building in the sense of preserving and nurturing is not making anything.
>
> (Heidegger, 2001, 145)

Back to building and dwelling. Perhaps dwelling and building are related as ends and means. Mortals build so they can dwell. My aim as a teacher is to make it possible for students to learn. I began to think about the idea of teaching and learning as the *thing* at the centre of the study. As I have said, the *thing* locates and gathers the fourfold. Building as preserving and nurturing resonates with my teaching. I want the students to find themselves in their own way. I try and create a space for that. I was intrigued; the fourfold spoke to a connectedness between things that gives a *thing* its meaning. The *thing*, phenomenon at the centre of my study is teaching and learning as relating. Heidegger uses tangible objects such as jug and bridge as examples of the fourfold. My study uses the fourfold to express the thing of teaching and learning as relating.

The process itself involved dwelling with the data, staying close, allowing the fourfold to show itself. I needed to be patient and allow my writing to show me the way. It is easy to get lost in Heidegger's philosophical writing. Philosophy can be seductive, but it is important to remember that I am a researcher using the philosophy of Heidegger to shine a light on the phenomenon I am studying. I cannot replicate philosophy. My task is to use philosophy to unpack how I learn as I teach, to weave these ideas into my thinking as I dwell with the data. The ongoing dwelling and staying with a willingness to be open to what would be revealed eventually bore fruit, but it took time and a lot of reading and reflecting.

One day after a visit to the art gallery, my visual creativity was re-aroused, and I started drawing diagrams as well as writing notes. Here is an example of writing in my journal about a moment of clearing that helped me find my way:

> All my writing so far is about finding space, dwelling, being open, negative capability (facing the here and now with an open mind). On the other hand, there is what one learns at teachers' college and then meeting the requirements of the university; however, for me the key is to stay in these spaces. How do I structure this? I could call one chapter preparation, enframing.

This journal entry marks the beginning of what would become the element *negotiated frame*. This was the element that was the last to fall into place. After writing this entry, I searched my emerging themes. I realised that I had been struggling to find a place for "culture and difference," a theme that was very present in Aotearoa, New Zealand. I had interviewed a rōpū (group) of Māori graduates from the Psychotherapy training. It became clear from the interview that the indigenous approach to teaching and learning was much more teacher centred. Māori and other minority groups felt othered by the dominant discourse. This naturally belongs with what is outside of my control and yet is part of the world I live in. Another important theme that fitted into the *negotiated frame* was how the teaching and learning process was enclosed by the university structures. What became clear as I was grappling with an earlier version of Figure 8.2 was that it is the sky that encloses the earth. The earth needs a medium through which it can appear. So, there needs to be an element that represents that which is beyond my control and which needs to be negotiated, like the weather. Thus, the *negotiated frame* as one of the elements was born. Overall the *negotiated frame* reflects the context of the teaching and learning situation. The frame is the underlying structure of the teaching event. Negotiation is the process that a teacher takes on in relation to all of that which is out of her control. It is exciting when the connection between the different themes arising from the analysis of the transcripts begins to unfold. Suddenly I saw that all my notes and writing about the interrelationship between appropriately using the university structures and my own approach to teaching fitted with Heidegger's thinking about technology (Heidegger, 1993). Technology stands for the part of the teaching that relates to the mechanised and measurable, for example, learning outcomes. Heidegger uses the phrase "*releasement towards things*" (Heidegger, 1966, 54) to describe a process whereby humans are able to use technology to support us, while also preventing technology diminishing our humanness. He saw technology as a part of Dasein because, after all, humanity has created all technology. "Releasement towards things" became the first sub-element of the *negotiated frame*. It began to make sense that the sub-elements folded into the fourfold structure just as the elements did. While I have unpacked all these elements and sub-elements (see Figure 8.2 for a complete overview), they all can be happening at once. The complexity that I have created reflects the doctoral process, the detail of moment-by-moment experiences. The beauty of the fourfold is that by being present to experience in a moment, any moment one enters through dwelling into the fourfold, touching its essence and thus making good use of the thing whatever it is. In the case of my study, the thing is teaching and learning as relating, involving engagement through *dwelling, negotiating the frame* (the context), *way-making* by taking action in relationship, and *learning from* my own experience in relation to those I am teaching and learning with. Next, I will give two examples of data from my thesis and a brief summary of how they relate to the elements of the fourfold.[4]

## Two examples

Through the ongoing hermeneutic process, I wrote my first findings chapter called "Learning to dwell." It flowed well. It felt correct, and yet I knew I did not have the full picture. I noted that when Heidegger talked about the fourfold, he always started with the earth. Nevertheless, the links to the fourfold were still not fully evident to me. The teacher's attention on relation-with-self is the expression of *learning to dwell*. The teacher's task is to be grounded in her own knowledge and yet "open" to the here and now, capable of "*letting the mind be a thoroughfare*" (Keats, 1891/1925, 1007), and ensuring she "*creates an open space*" for herself. This prepares me, the teacher, to facilitate and maintain a mood in the classroom that enables the students to learn. *Learning to dwell* means being able to bear the feelings that are aroused and to stay with oneself until the meaning arises from within. Here is an example. It is a memory I wrote in my journal that I was reminded of in an interview.

> I remember in the second year of teaching at the Uni, getting excited about the ideas, and all the psychotherapy articles I could use to teach. One I remember was when I was teaching the oedipus complex and gender issues to 2nd year Masters students. I tried to include a huge range of papers and I read them all. Naturally the students didn't. What I was confronted with in the classroom was the reality of who the students were. There was a strong representation of gay and lesbian students and they were very challenging about the Freudian theory. I can remember the recognition of, "this is what it is all about, I need to work with their views too". One part of me was curious and another part of me was a bit anxious, understanding that I had something to learn here. I discovered that I needed to find a way to be with their thinking and take it on board without dropping all of my own thinking. They had their own ideas and my task was to find a way to facilitate thinking about the

different ideas together and make the link to experience and especially to practice. I loved that class. They taught me a lot.

This story reveals the sub-element of "openness" (my noting and reflecting on the experience in the classroom), "letting the mind be a thoroughfare" (allowing the students to have an impact on me and willingness to recognise where they were coming from), and "creating space" (finding a way to facilitate thinking about different ideas together). "Openness" is implicit in my own willingness to be a learner and open to what the students bring to the teaching space. The quote, *"Letting the mind be a thoroughfare"* is from Keats (1891/1925). My interpretation of this is that having the mind as a thoroughfare is allowing oneself to be present and for thoughts to move freely without attachment so that the meaning that arises comes from a combination of who I am, the students and the context. Heidegger (2001, 6) states, *"We never come to thoughts. They come to us."* I think for this to occur, we need to learn to dwell, which Heidegger defined thus.

> It is enough if we dwell on what lies close and meditate on what is closest; upon that which concerns us, each one of us, here and now; here on this patch of home ground; now, in the present hour of history.
>
> (Heidegger, 1966, 47)

Reflecting on this now, it became obvious that *learning to dwell* represents part of the fourfold, earth which is my starting place from before teaching starts and ongoingly through the teaching year.

The next chapter to emerge was *way-making* – as bringing another to learning. That chapter mapped the journey of teaching and learning for me and for my students over a year. The word way comes from Old English *weg* meaning road, path (Etymonline.com), while make comes from Old English *macian*, which means to give being to, give form or character to, bring into existence, to build. This links to Heidegger's words, *"The way is such, it lets us reach what concerns and summons us"* (1971, 91). When Heidegger speaks of the way to language, he questions the way we use language and shows us through his questioning his own way-making. He says, *"Such way-making brings language (the essence of language) as language (the saying) to language (to the resounding word)."* (Heidegger, 1993, 418). He adds, *"… the way to language … becomes possible and necessary only by virtue of the way proper, the way-making movement of propriation[5] and usage"* (Heidegger, 1993, 419). Heidegger uses the term way-making to unpack the use of language, stressing the importance of finding the correct horizon through which to view our event. *Way-making* indicates movement and, in the example below is revealed through feeling the flow of the combination of myself, the material, and the students, as we work together. *Way-making* represents mortals as part of the fourfold. The link is to the students who come for a while and then leave, whose existence in my teaching and learning experience is always temporary. The students' task is to learn, which in my view requires a capacity to dwell and facilitates a possibility of being true to oneself.

The following vignette illustrates the element *way-making*, captured when I was interviewed about a particular teaching experience:

> It was assessment day. The students were presenting their piece of verbatim recording with an introduction, brief case outline and discussion. After the assessments, I let them know what they did well and offered critique. As I walked away from the classroom, I had this sudden clunk inside as I remembered one of the conversations in that session. One of the students had said how hard she could be on herself and how that was a real difficulty for her. I had replied, "Yes, it is really important to discriminate between using your critique and being reflexive and on the other hand, being hard on yourself". The clunk moment came when I heard my voice and noticed that my tone was critical and dismissive. My words were ok, it was something in the mood that felt difficult. I was able to unpack the process of it and understand what had happened – from my perspective. In the next session I let the students know that I had reflected on my response to them in the feedback session and recognised my critical tone. We discussed this for a while and then I resumed teaching this last session of the day. Next morning the students were still in an irritable, uncomfortable mood. What emerged in the check-in session after the poem was that they were upset with my comment in the feedback. I had said that I was disappointed that in their presentations they had left so little time for discussion. They told me they too were disappointed that in the final session of the day I had finished too late and didn't give the students time for a check out. I could see their point. I said, "Yes, you are correct". At some stage I said, "It is interesting to see how we all became infected by the assessment process this time". We spent some time reflecting together on our varied experiences of the day before. After this we got on with the work of the day. At the end of this day when we were checking out there was a story from a student who today had become aware of how "rugged up"[6] she was. She recognised that she felt self-protective and had needed the extra warmth her partner's clothes provided because she was carrying her memory of the intensely painful experience of writing her case-study in the psychotherapy programme some years ago. She said that somehow yesterday she had re-entered that zone and felt a need to protect herself and had needed that extra warmth and the experience of being together with the class and with me and that today she had felt different. She had appreciated the process of the teaching. It had helped her learn and create a new experience for herself. [*Interview 13*]

My process, as teacher, of recognising and unpacking the mood of the experience in the classroom, is part of how I "hold" the class. It is my commitment to being reflexive, or befindlichkeit translated by Gendlin (1978–1979) as how-you-areness or self finding. It creates an atmosphere of trust and safety. Allowing a space for each individual to bring their story requires ongoing "holding." This is done partly through beginning the day or session by offering a poem and then asking for their associations. This provides the possibility of students moving their awareness from calculative to meditative thinking. The end of the day or session is another opportunity to create a space for reflection, to review learning, and, as the example above shows, "learning to think" and "learn from experience" (sub-element of *learning from*).

The capacity to disagree with each other, to reveal the lack of agreement, is only possible if the students feel safe to be themselves. I continually reflect back the students' experience and note my own. I name the acceptance of different perspectives. What is revealed through the experience of "dissonance" in me, and in the students was that we were upset about different moments. The "holding" continues as we stay with the hermeneutics-of-mood (to represent the back and forth of sifting through our different responses together). "*Mood ... is not a mere accompaniment to being-in-the-world. It discloses the world, reveals our thrownness into it, and enables us to respond to beings within it*" (Inwood, 1999, 132). At the same time, we got on with the task of teaching and learning. There is a symmetry between the content we are focusing on and the process that is going on in the classroom. The curriculum is used as a resource rather than the sole focus of the learning.

*Mitdasein* literally means "being-with" each other as a class. In my thesis, this is called "Using intersubjective space." "The world of Dasein is a with-world [*Mitwelt*]. Being-in is *being-with* Others. Their Being-in-themselves within-the-world is *Dasein-with* [*Mitdasein*]" (Heidegger, 2008, 155). Heidegger has been critiqued for his focus on subjectivity rather than intersubjectivity (O'Brien, 2014). I am aware that I have interpreted Heidegger based on my own perspective that Dasein is firmly a self + world – that one is already always centred in the context of the social world where others are active in their engagement. The social world is inseparable from the world of Dasein. Another way of articulating *mitdasein* is co-openness. Sheehan (2001, 200) says, "*This co-openness is also the basis for all forms of interpersonal togetherness.*" Thus, *mitdasein* in my classroom means sharing our different points of view with each other. Doing this facilitates the capacity for "learning to think." This is evident in the transcript with the student who describes herself as "rugged up." She questions her fore-structure and is able to express her discomfort and resolution of that discomfort. Heidegger offers the view that way-making is on the path towards ourselves, not a singular self (Heidegger, 2001). So, while I tell the story of one, in particular, all have their own journey in this vignette.

*Learning from* is the last theme to emerge from my data and relates to developing the capacity to think. In Heideggerian terms, this means being open. Heidegger describes the core aspects of meditative thinking as being releasement towards things and openness to the mystery, requiring a willingness to engage in "*persistent, courageous thinking*" (Heidegger, 1966, 57). Given the hiddenness of Being and the ongoing unknownness accompanying the query "what is called thinking," releasement towards things involves surrendering to experience as much as possible, "reflecting" on what is known and even more on what cannot be known, while at the same time staying grounded and open. I interpret this to mean letting be while I dwell on what is my task at this moment. I imagine that I will only ever get close to releasement towards things and openness to the mystery (that which cannot yet be seen, understood, heard, or spoken but perhaps which is sensed in some way). As is evident from the example above, the teacher and the student need to be reflexive and willing to be true to themselves when speaking. It is especially hard with a large class or a class of students who do not know each other. My study illustrates the usefulness of engaging with each other, to bring the voices of each person in the class to facilitate "learning from experience," and to reflect what Heidegger calls meditative thinking.

## And finally

I think that writing a doctoral thesis using hermeneutic phenomenology requires an intricate balance between openness and structure. I needed to be open to the data, open to the point of expanding my horizon beyond what I know and what I know that I do not know I know. Alongside that openness, I also needed some way of organising the material, my analysis and the process of my interpretations as it unfolded. My journals provided that resource, organised by time, always recording what I was reading and thinking about.

Psychoanalytic theory and Heidegger concur in the need to "*expose [the] inner structural skeleton [of one's history]*" (Harman, 2007, 59). For Heidegger this addresses the historical structure of Dasein which locks humans into interpreting the world in the same way others do. My own history and training helped me to be present to my own processes, to be reflective and open to how I was being. Choosing a self-study (hermeneutics of self) was challenging. It brought up fears of being solipsistic and of being overexposed. On the other hand, it allowed me as a researcher with my participants to explore and question the subtle variations in the teaching and learning process. I think another factor that made it possible to embark on this arduous approach to research was that I had been a psychotherapist and teacher of psychotherapy for many years. My own robustness was an important resource for this method.

In this chapter, I have shown how I used dwelling in the fourfold as a structure for the themes that emerge in my thesis, drawing on the philosophy of Heidegger and his phenomenological hermeneutic research approach. The process of this is convoluted and required me to surrender my need to know. That was an interesting process for me because there was a sense in which I already knew how to do that. Clearly, there were ways of surrendering my attachment to certain types of knowledge (ontic thinking) I had not explored yet. I learned that we always create structures, it is part of being human, of Dasein. The fourfold is a set of structures that underpin human existence when humanity can existentially dwell, that is, live with acceptance and understanding of our thrownness. What helped me in this research endeavour was to read Heidegger, to dwell with the data and to journal. It was to trust that insight would come, in its own way, in its own time. It was to know that even with the thesis examined, even with this chapter written, the thinking goes on. In another sense, the fourfold needs to gather in any thesis for the thing to be revealed, for the thing at the centre of any thesis to be unconcealed. Heidegger's use of the concept *thing* helps us to remember that no-thing is fixed, the meaning is created by how we use it.

## Notes

1. Heidegger (2008, 32) says that being ontological implies an understanding of being. Harman (2007, 176) succinctly states that ontic refers to a particular being while ontological refers to being itself. Another useful source in attempting to understand the difference between Ontic and ontological is Gendlin (1978/9, 11) as follows, "Heidegger uses the word "ontic" for ordinary assertions of anything, and the word "ontological" for the understanding of the kind of being of anything."
2. An object can be touched and seen, its outside appearance is what matters. A thing has an essence. An object is present-to-hand while a thing exists in its own right. Harman (2009, 293) suggests that thing could be said to be absent-at-hand. This is because a thing stands independently of its production, saying how it was made does not reveal what it is.
3. From this point onward, I am at times using the elements and sub-elements that revealed themselves in my data. The elements will be underlined and the sub-elements will have single brackets around them.
4. Perhaps it is important to note here that these transcripts and my thinking about them described here form only a small portion of the material I used to create my fourfold.
5. Propriation is a translation of ereignis and another word for event. Braver (2009, 113) describes propriation thus, "propriation is and only is the event of our ability to perceive, think, and speak about beings, their intellible presence to us."
6. Rugged up is a New Zealand term that means to wrap up.

## References

Braver, L. 2009. *Heidegger's later writings: A reader's guide*. London: Continuum.

Brownell, P. 2016. "Contemporary gestalt therapy." *Contemporary theory and practice in counseling and psychotherapy*, edited by H. E. A. Tinsley, S. H. Lease and N. S. G. Wiersma, 407–433. New York, NY: Sage, Ebook.

Falkenstrom, F. 2007. "The psychodynamics of self-observation." *Psychoanalytic Dialogues* 17 (4): 551–574. https://doi.org/10.1080/10481880701487318

Fleck, K., E. Smythe, and J. Hitchens. 2011. "Hermeneutics of self as a research approach." *International Journal of Qualitative Methods* 10 (1): 14–29. https://doi.org/10.1177/160940691101000102

Freud, S. 1913. "On beginning the treatment (further recommendations on the technique of psycho-analysis 1)." *The standard edition of the complete psychological works of Sigmund Freud, Volume XII (1911–1913): The case of Schreber, papers on technique and other works, 121–144*, edited by J. Strachey. London: Hogarth Press. 1953.

Gendlin, E. 1978–1979. "Befindlichkeit: Heidegger and the philosophy of psychology." *Review of Existential Psychology and Psychiatry: Heidegger and Psychology* XVI (1–3): 43–71.

Harman, G. 2007. *Heidegger explained: From phenomenon to things*. Chicago, IL: Open Court.

Harman, G. 2009. "Dwelling with the fourfold." *Space and Culture* 12 (3): 292–302. https://doi.org/10.1177/1206331209337080

Heidegger, M. 1966. *Discourse on thinking*. Translated by J. Anderson and E. H. Freund. New York, NY: Harper Perennial. 1959.

Heidegger, M. 1971. *On the way to language*. Translated by P. D. Hertz. San Francisco, CA: HarperCollins. 1959.

Heidegger, M. 1993. *Martin Heidegger: Basic writings*. Translated by D. F. Krell. 2nd ed. New York, NY: Harper Collins. 1977.

Heidegger, M. 1998. *Pathmarks*, edited by W. McNeil. New York, NY: Cambridge University Press.

Heidegger, M. 2001. *Poetry, language, thought*. Translated by A. Hofstadter. New York, NY: Harper Collins. 1971.

Heidegger, M. 2008. *Being and time*. Translated by J. Macquarrie and E. Robinson. 7th ed. New York, NY: Harper and Row. Reprint, 2008. 1962.

Heidegger, M. 2012. *Bremen and Freiburg lectures: Insight into that which is and basic principles of thinking*. Translated by A. J. Mitchell. Bloomington, IN: Indiana University Press. 1994.

Inwood, M. 1999. *A Heidegger dictionary*. Oxford, UK: Blackwell.

Keats, J. 1925. *Letters of John Keats to his family and friends*, edited by S. Colvin. London, England: Macmillan and Co. Ltd. 1891.

Mitchell, A. J. 2015. *The fourfold: Reading the later Heidegger*. Evanston, IL: Northwestern University Press.

O'Brien, M. 2014. "Leaping ahead of Heidegger: Subjectivity and intersubjectivity in Being and Time." *International Journal of Philosophical Studies* 22 (4): 534–551. https://doi.org/10.1080/09672559.2014.948719

Sheehan, T. 2001. "A paradigm shift in Heidegger research." *Continental Philosophy Review* 34: 183–202.

Solomon, M. 2014. "Reverie and reflection: Thinking in the marrowbone." *Ata: Journal of Psychotherapy Aotearoa New Zealand* 18 (1): 11–21. https://doi.org/10.9791/ajpanz.2014.02

Solomon, M. 2017. *"Teaching and learning as relating: A transformational experience."* Doctor of Health Science, Psychotherapy, AUT.

Young, J. 2002. *Heidegger's later philosophy*. New York, NY: Cambridge University Press.

# 9 Working with phenomenon

## Just keep swimming

*Christine Edwards*

## Abstract

Working with hermeneutic phenomenology reminds me of the story Finding Nemo and Dory's search for Nemo into the dark unknown. Often lost, not knowing where to look next, Dory "just keeps on swimming," following her instincts and trusting she will find Nemo. My search to uncover shared meanings of the phenomenological nature of "care" in the context of Human Resource Management in higher education took me on a similar journey into the unknown. Often the journey felt impossible. Often, I felt trapped, stuck, looking "outside there" for answers. The answers were never where I "looked." When I trusted my own instincts with the courage to "let go" and allow the phenomenon to guide me, glimpses of understanding shone through the darkness. My journey began with my own stories of care to reveal my pre-understandings of the phenomenon. Then, I interviewed others to reveal their stories. I searched for meaning in their stories, constantly returning to the phenomenon, questioning and thinking, "what is mattering?" and "what is being revealed?" I became a solicitous eyewitness to the lived experience of "care." New insights brought to light the remarkable in the unremarkable. The aesthetic use of language allowed me to create a space where my thoughts were free to play and wonder and where the ontological meanings of the phenomenon of "care" were revealed.

## My story

I was experiencing a very difficult time in my life. I was worried, distressed, things seemed hopeless. I could see no way out. I did not know what I was to do. I recall my teenage daughter saying to me in a very matter of fact way, 'just keep swimming'. Puzzled I asked her, 'what do you mean?' 'Just keep swimming', she repeated. 'You know, like Dory in the movie Finding Nemo when all seemed lost, she just kept swimming'. I laughed. I remembered the scene in the movie very clearly. Dory and Marvin (Nemo's Dad) were journeying down into the deepest, darkest part of the ocean looking for the elusive Nemo. Marvin was fearful of the dark and of the unknown and wanted to give up. But Dory, unaware of the dangers and embracing the darkness, urged Marvin on by singing, *just keep swimming, just keep swimming*. It worked. I just kept swimming my way through the dark unknown. Working with phenomenon to research the lived-experience I learned to embrace the dark corners of the unknown. I learned, even in the most difficult moments to just keep

DOI: 10.4324/9781003081661-9

swimming, to trust the understandings "would come" and eventually a path to new understandings would present itself as glimpses of light in the dark. The wisdom of my daughter (and Dory) is a powerful reminder. Sometimes you just have to have blind faith that things will work out and keep on ongoing despite not knowing what lies ahead and just keep swimming.

My journey began with my own experiences of care in my role as a Director of Human Resources. I experienced the tears, the frustrations and the joys that were part of the daily difficulties of balancing the constant economic imperative with my values and the needs and well-being of staff. I was increasingly concerned with decisions and policymaking in Human Resource Management (HRM) in higher education that privileged the science of productivity over the art of human-well-being. I left my role disillusioned, feeling physically ill and mentally exhausted wondering, does it have to be like this? Have we learned that good management is never to be corrupted by human kindness and compassion? Is it OK to mask human emotions? Is it OK for people to feel insecure, manipulated and left searching for meaning in their work? Is this the new normal in which care is taken-for-granted? I wondered about understandings of care and the impact of dominant economic rationalist values in HRM on people in universities. This led me to explore ontological understandings of care: "*to do justice to everyday experience, to evoke what it is to be human*" working in higher education (Finlay 2011, 3).

Thus, I began my search to uncover new understandings and shared meanings of the phenomenon of care in the context of HRM in higher education. My search took me into a dark unknown. Often the journey felt impossible. Often, I felt trapped, stuck, looking for answers "out there." But the answers were never where I "looked." I found there are no answers, only new understandings. And when I trusted in my own instincts with the courage to "let go" and allow the phenomenon to guide me, only then did glimpses of new understanding shine through the darkness.

## Revealing the remarkable in the unremarkable

Phenomenology is a search to recover a "*deeper understanding of the nature of meaning of our everyday lives*" (van Manen 1990, 9) and allow meanings to be seen anew. In Heidegger's (1962) view, these understandings are pre-reflective and *a priori*,[1] showing the taken-for-grantedness of our everyday experience. van Manen (1990) proposes that "*a real understanding of phenomenology can only be accomplished by actively doing it*" (8). My experience of working with the phenomenon, like Dory in her search for Nemo, was not a case of following a simple step-by-step path. Like Dory, most of the time, I had no idea what lay ahead. I had to follow my instinct and trust the phenomenon to guide me. As van Manen (1990, 29) suggested, the path to researching the lived experience could not "*be determined by fixed signposts.*" My path or method was conceived along the way in response to what was "at hand" (29).

Gadamer (2013) uses the metaphor of walking along a path in a forest that is taken-for-granted to describe the journey of re-covering meaning in our lived

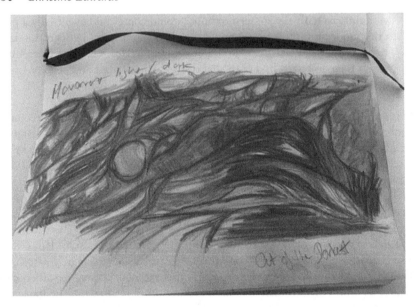

*Figure 9.1* My Journey of Re-covering Meaning

experiences. My path was more like swimming in an ocean exposed to the ebbs and flows of the tides and currents at any moment (Figure 9.1). I resided and experienced the research journey as a participant and not as a passive observer (Giles 2008; Smythe et al. 2008; van Manen 1990).

At times it was an arduous journey. Like Dory and Marvin in their search for the elusive Nemo, out of the dangers of the unknown grew new strengths and the deliverance of new understandings. At the beginning of the search, without being able to grasp onto the certainty of pre-defined steps, I often felt insecure. I stepped outside the research phenomenon, returning to a way of thinking and being I was comfortable with. I found myself looking for answers out there rather than allowing new possibilities to emerge through introspection and contemplation.

While working with a phenomenon may seem unmethodological, *"it is not a process of do whatever you like"* (Smythe et al. 2008, 1389). This was not simply a matter of sitting back and "navel gazing." On the contrary, I found the challenge was staying *in* the search with a contemplative intensity, knowing that that which is most essential to us withdraws from us (Gadamer 2013; Heidegger 1962). As van Manen (1990) suggests, the phenomenological path requires scholarship as the researcher becomes a *"sensitive observer of the subtleties of everyday life and an avid reader of relevant text … humanities, history, philosophy, anthropology and the social sciences as they pertain to his or her domain of interest"* (29).

Faithfully giving into and residing in the search, I found as I moved through and engaged with the phenomenon and just kept swimming, living towards the phenomenon, I experienced the feeling of being in-play (Heidegger 1962). I understood my role as a researcher to make visible what is hidden. To bring to light the remarkable in unremarkable everyday experiences. I became a solicitous eyewitness to the ontological meanings and the taken-for-granted understandings in everyday lived experiences of care in HRM processes in universities. Free from *"the noise that tells us all that is already known"* I found myself in a *"space"* where my thoughts were free to play and wonder and where renewed insights came (Smythe et al. 2008, 1391). Even though, at times working phenomenologically was a journey of trepidation, it was always a journey of wonderment and awe. I often amazed myself as the deepening connection with my work was revealed in the salvation of trusting my intuition, acknowledging feelings without having to rationalise them, and the serendipity of those moments when new possibilities appeared. I discovered *"the objectivity of [my] work was secured in the deepened awareness of its subjectivity"* (Romanyshyn 2013, 169). From my experience in working with phenomenon, I came to understand the *"way of being-phenomenological"* cannot be forced or induced, it *"comes"* (Smythe et al. 2008, 1394).

## Working with phenomenon: guided by existential philosophers who light the way

Working with phenomenon is *"found within the wider philosophical underpinnings"* (Ehrich 1999, 20). Phenomenological practice is sound when it is allied to a phenomenological philosophy (of which I found there were many) (Ehrich 1999; Finlay 2012). I chose the works of existential philosophers, Heidegger and Gadamer to illuminate understandings in my study.

The writings of Heidegger and Gadamer were the shining lights to reveal the taken-for-granted understandings of the nature of care in HRM in Higher Education. I chose the existential phenomenological path because it is concerned with the existence of being and upholds that experience as the principal interest of phenomenology (Ehrich 1999). I chose Heidegger's philosophical understandings of how it is to be because *"for Heidegger, ontology, phenomenology, hermeneutics and language are brought together in a 'lived-experience'"* (Giles 2008, 64).

Gadamer developed Heidegger's ideas into a practical way of working phenomenologically. Gadamer (2013) believed the preoccupation with (objective) method or technique is antithetical to the spirit of human science scholarship. Gadamer (2001) proposed ways to work phenomenologically with hermeneutics at its core: *"descriptively, creatively-intuitively, and in a concretizing manner"* (113). In following this philosophy, my search was a faithful (and always fateful) journey of playful wondering, thinking and sense-making where I was immersed in a cycle of disciplined and committed reading, writing and dialogue (Smythe et al. 2008; van Manen 1990).

## The presence of Heidegger

In Heidegger's (1962) philosophy, hermeneutic phenomenology uncovers the mysteries, wonders and awe of the nature of Being in ways in which humans fulfil possibilities in the world into which they are born and inevitably die. All being is in Being (Heidegger 1962). The meaning of the phenomenon of care in the Heideggerian perspective can only be in *experiencing* care.

## Heidegger on Care

Heidegger's philosophy of phenomenology is ontological in that *"the most signifi-cant order of reality is meaning, not matter, and in which meaning is organised accord-ing to aesthetic principles instead of the principles of formal logic"* (Polkinghorne 1988, 159). The phenomenological/ontological search is life-giving as it returns to the experience of careing[2] of care, in all the messy, dynamic, unpredictable, astonishing, bewildering and ever emerging meaning.

Heidegger signals to the nature of phenomenon as something which is *"revealing and concealing, coming and going, present absent, (and) a thrownness"* (Moules et al. 2015, 23). In a Heideggerian understanding of phenomenon, the everydayness of "care" may be hidden. What might appear as "care" may not be care at all, or vice versa (Smythe 2003). The hermeneutic challenge in interpreting the nature of the phenomenon in my inquiry was to shine a light to reveal that which is unseen in the everyday experience of care in HRM practice in higher education.

Care is at the centre of Heidegger's (1962) philosophy. Heidegger used the word care at a deepening ontological level to describe the essence of Dasein (Gelven 1989). Not to be confused with ontic understandings of care and caring, for Heidegger, care *"accounts for the unity, authenticity and totality of the self, that is, of Dasein"* (Reich 1995, 7). Dasein is care. Heidegger (1962) explains the tendency of Dasein to turn away from its own authentic being, and in seeking security in the crowd, limit its way of being to what others think, and behave in accordance with public opinion (the They) (also discussed by Liz and Deb, Chapter 2, Lesley Kay, Chapter 5 and Jean, Chapter 11).

As in Roman mythology, care in Heidegger's philosophy has dual meanings of anxiety and solicitude, representing two conflicting, fundamental possibilities in everyday experience. Sorge, anxious, worrisome care represents the struggle for survival and status approval among fellow human beings. Fürsorge, solicitous care or "caring for" represents attending to, nurturing, caring for the Earth and for others. Both care as anxiety and care as solicitude are experienced in the everyday world of being. Worrisome or troubling care may move us to escape and solicitous care can open us to possibilities (Reich 1995).

Heidegger (1962) made the distinction between "taking care of" in the sense of supplying to the needs of others, Besorgen, and Fürsorgen, "caring for." Dasein, that is, essentially related to others, enters the world of others by way of care as Besorgen and care as Fürsorgen. Heidegger's insights on Sorge, Fürsorge, Besorgen and Dasein formed the philosophical foundations for the notions of care devel-oped in coming to understandings of care in HRM in higher education.

## The presence of Hans-Georg Gadamer

Gadamer's work maintained hermeneutics at the centre of his philosophy. Building upon linguistic and ontological themes from Heidegger, Gadamer (2013) extended the idea of philosophical hermeneutics. Gadamer believed that to understand something is to find a way of applying it to our own circumstances and testing our understandings against our own pre-conceptions. In this way, "application" can only be viewed as integral to understanding human beings and *"never (as) an add-on to that which has already been understood"* (Nixon 2017, 53). Rather than provide a method or set of rules to apply to the search for understandings, Gadamer offers ways of being in the search and ways to ponder and question, beginning with the unique culturally and historically formed consciousness of the researcher, *"to light an interpretation that has revelatory power"* (Gadamer 2001, 42; Nixon 2017). Because each researcher brings to the search their own unique formed consciousness, the phenomenon and the context is specified, and understanding is always a unique possibility.

## Hermeneutic circling: faith in the Darkest

In line with Gadamer's writings towards "living language" and moving towards understanding as the distinguishing character of language, the hermeneutic circle describes this movement as present understanding or prejudice interacting with and moving into, new understandings (Moules et al. 2015). Heidegger (1962) referred to the hermeneutic circle to explain the interaction between part and whole, the back and forth understanding of Dasein. Gadamer (2013) refers to the circular movement as vital to recovering meanings, *"this circle is constantly expanding, since the concept of the world is relative, and being integrated in ever larger contexts always affects the understanding of the individual parts"* (196).

I expressed my experience of the hermeneutic circle as the dynamic movement between light and dark in this poem.

> The Light of meaning hovers there
> In the Darkest, some nearby thought coming forth
> Illuminates a tiny part of my mind
> Have Faith in the Darkest
> Another turn, another ephemeral moment, dark and then light
> A light muted, fleeting. It shines afresh,
> Light in the shadows, quivers, streaks my mindfulness
> Only to fade, and disappear.
> I turn once again toward the Darkest.
> For the Light, swallowed by the gloom of the Darkest smoulders,
> fades then glows, grows
> Have faith in the Darkest. *Just keep swimming.* The Light will come.

Some commentators refer to the hermeneutic spiral signifying an imaginal approach, that is, the poetics of research and its transcendent function between conscious and unconscious (Romanyshyn 2013). According to Romanyshyn (2013), spiralling represents a deepening engagement between the researcher and their interpretive work *"expressed in dreams, intuitions, feelings, symptoms, and synchronicities"* (216). Both Heidegger and Gadamer emphasise the aesthetic or poetic use of language to move towards meaning, unfolding and deepening within and out of present meanings in the presence of the researcher with all their traditions, both conscious and unconscious. Rich within the heritage of Hermes that *"brings the message of destiny*" (Heidegger 1962, as cited in Romanyshyn 2013, 220), hermeneutic turning, circling and/or spiralling is an ongoing movement as the language of description of what the phenomenon "*is*" disappears and the ontological nature is revealed in the language of deepening understanding of the "*isness*" or essence of its meaning. Once again, I turned to poetry to express my own experience of hermeneutic circle as follows.

> Every lock is its key.
> Every shadow is its Light.
> In the whirlpool of my mind, no torpid loops.
> An illuminating Light, from the deep,
> Straining, revealing that which is unseen.
> Then sublimity, the moment one thing is about to become something else,
> Dark into Light

Understandings often came to me, in what seemed to be my darkest moments, as illuminating flashes appearing and disappearing. As Dick (1992) says, "*just when the darkness seems to have smothered all, to be truly transcendent, the new seeds of light are reborn*" (95).

## Shaping the inquiry

The broader phenomenological research community had a significant influence on me and my search. After attending an international conference on interpretive phenomenology, I had a sense of feeling at home with a way of thinking and a way of being in research that did not attempt to put ideas or people into tight compartments. The opening address sets the scene.

> We are not going to get to the point.
> We are not going to point at …
> We are going to point to …
> (Giles 2016)

By the end of the conference, I found myself falling into a phenomenological way of being. I scribbled the following poem to express my sense of freedom and possibility as I stood poised, ready to begin my own journey working with phenomenon.

> The 'ing' ing of living
> The 'is' ness of is
> The 'all in' ness of self and others
> Hope in the unseen
> Grace and fellowship in the uncovered life
> Possibilities in the glimmering moments in the darkened room

Possible research questions began to form as I pondered lived experiences in higher education and identifying an underlying phenomenon:

- How is the taken-for-granted, accepted ways of being an employee lived out?
- How is the presence of a sense of void[3] experienced in the everyday work life within universities?

- How are care, compassion, humility and even hope experienced in the workplace?
- How is care, as a phenomenon of the existential nature of being human, experienced in workplace relationships in higher education?

The research question for this inquiry was finally shaped as, "*What is the ontological nature of the phenomenon of 'care' as experienced in HRM in higher education?*"

## Capturing thoughts and feelings along the way

From the outset, I kept a journal of conversations, teaching notes, quotations, interactions and reflections on care. As I progressed, thoughts and insights would come and go at all times and places, in the car, on the bus, in unrelated conversations. Thoughts found me. Often thoughts would come, not quite fully formed, and then disappear, only to reappear in a different form. I was drawn to these thoughts as if they were signposts, a pointer, pointing in that moment "*at something which has not, not yet, been transposed into the language of [our] speech*" (Heidegger 1968, 18; Polkinghorne 1989).

I kept my journal and a pen with me to capture these as they appeared or improvised by recording thoughts on my phone, scraps of paper and post-it notes. Journaling provided a "memoir" of my journey and references of my understandings to reflect upon as they appeared and then disappeared.

## Being interviewed myself

Uncovering the ontological nature that exists in human experiences of the phenomenon of care started with gathering a collection of experiential textual descriptions of care in universities in the form of stories (Polkinghorne 1989). The first stories I gathered were stories of my own experiences. Because we are, as Gadamer (1998) said, "*historical creatures, we are always on the inside of the history that we are striving to understand*" (28), it was necessary, for me as the researcher, to first acknowledge my own prejudices. Therefore, I was interviewed as a starting point for "*the retrieval of any prejudices that is naively covered over*"[4] (Diekelmann 2005, 23) (also see Chapter 2).

Reflecting upon my first experience of a hermeneutic interview, I was surprised by the ease with which I shared my stories. It was then I understood the importance for the interviewer to be interested and engaged as we fell "*into conversation*" (Gadamer 2013, 401). Together we reviewed the interview questions and notes. I noticed there were a few "prepared" questions. However, I could see that I was only asked one of the prepared questions. Other questions were asked in response to my answers. In reviewing the interviewer's notes, I saw the ways in which one word followed another and the turnings as the interviewer allowed me to progress down a path with neither of us knowing what will "*come out of a conversation*" (Gadamer 2013, 401). What struck me was how the initial question opened up the conversation, as comments pointed to more questions and probes, allowing my story to lead and take its own course and reach its own conclusion (Gadamer 2013). The experience appreciably changed my perspective of care. Speaking freely and out loud about my experience of care gave me a sense of satisfaction and relief that I had been heard. The new insights I gained were the basis of many discussions over the following weeks and the subject of my journaling.

My stories became the text for exploring the prejudices and assumptions I held in relation to the phenomenon of care. These stories raised my awareness of my own experiences of the phenomenon, providing *"clues for orientating [myself] to the phenomenon and thus to all other stages of phenomenological research"* (van Manen 1990, 57). According to Gadamer (2013, 282), it is important to be open to the other while recognising our own biases in order to *"be aware of one's own biases, so that the text can present itself in all its otherness and thus assert its own truth against one's own fore-meanings."* Interpretation and understanding always occur based on our own historical context; our prior experiences influence our own fore-meaning. Listening to, reading and re-reading my own stories of care as a daughter, mother, employee and manager helped to reveal my own fore-meanings or pre-understandings. These revelations enabled me to understand the meanings in the stories of another with a renewed perspective.

### Locating other storytellers

The participants in this inquiry were employed in the Schools of Education from two universities in Adelaide, Australia. The participants had experienced the phenomenon of care from working within or working with HR policies and practices in their university. The different positions, roles or levels of the participants in the university were not specified in the recruitment and selection process. As phenomenology derives meaning from the experiences *"without a prescribed viewpoint of power or gender"* (Smythe 2012, 6), the participants' job role or position in the university was not important; it was their experience that was essential.

Participants were identified using a snowball sampling technique.[5] In snowball or purposeful sampling, people are selected because they are information rich and offer useful manifestations of the phenomenon (Patton 2002). Snowballing identifies an initial participant who then provides the names of other possible participants. This continues to snowball, opening prospects for expanding connections of contact and inquiry. Snowball sampling takes advantage of the social networks of identified participants, which are used to provide an ever-increasing set of potential contacts (Atkinson and Flint 2004).

### Gathering the stories in conversation

Each participant was interviewed once. The purpose of the hermeneutic phenomenological interview was to gather thick descriptions of everyday experiences of care in HRM in higher education (van Manen 1990). Therefore, the interviews were largely unstructured and opened by asking participants to *Tell me about a time when* …. to draw out participants' stories of their experiences of care. A set of open-ended questions were formulated to evoke a broad storytelling of the participants' experiences. There was no mention of care in the initial interview questions. This was a deliberate approach to minimise the possibility that participants would theorise or attempt to describe *good* and *bad* care.

I was conscious not to *conduct* the interviews, as "*a genuine conversation is never one that we want to conduct*" (Gadamer 2013, 401). I engaged in a conversation by telling the participants a little about myself and asking them about themselves and their role in their institution. Most of the time, I did not need to use or refer to the questions I had prepared. It was clear participants had reflected upon their experiences prior to the interview. They had already thought of stories to tell and were eager to share them. So, I found myself falling with them into conversation, engaged and listening, occasionally seeking clarification or prompting for more.

## Uncovering thematic aspects

I transcribed the interviews and, as I did, re-experienced the participants' experiences. Then I read each transcript several times while the interpretive process began to identify the ontological meanings of the text and subtext. I listened to and read the transcripts, turning and re-turning to the text and my understandings, allowing phrases and statements that seemed "to matter" to the shared experiences of the phenomena to come forth (Smythe 2003; Smythe et al. 2008).

The interview transcripts provided a broad range of stories: textual descriptions of care. The stories were handled in a process similar to that outlined by Caelli (2001), Giles (2008) and Smythe et al. (2008) – transcribing the digital audio recording, reading the transcripts, reconstructing or crafting the stories in a chronological and/or logical order using the participants' words where possible. The crafted stories were returned to the participant to be approved for use in the interpretive stage of the inquiry. These crafted stories then formed the basis of an increasingly deepening interpretive and sense-making activity (Caelli 2001; Crowther et al. 2017).

## Working with the stories

Working with the phenomenon, I journeyed within the crafted stories in the space of disciplined thinking, writing and re-writing known as hermeneutic circling to guide my interpretation of essential meanings within the participants' experiences (Giles 2008; Smythe et al. 2008; van Manen 1990). I was always conscious of remembering care and keeping care alive in the search, as a fundamental attitude of phenomenology is that "*consciousness is not passive to the world*" (Jackson 2013, 85). Therefore, I constantly returned to the phenomenon, keeping care in mind, questioning and thinking, "*what matters?,*" "*what is being revealed?*" and "*how are my understandings increasing/developing from the story?*" (Smythe et al. 2008).

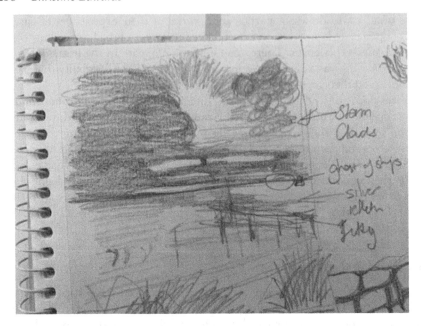

*Figure 9.2* Drawing to Express the Emergent Theme Safe at Home

I was mindful there is no right or wrong answer and knowing is always both knowing and not knowing. At the same time, I was conscious I was entrusted with these stories and my interpretations needed to be trustworthy. As I contemplated each story, I asked, "*have I let go of my own pre-understandings?*," "*am I open to new understandings without pre-judging?*," "*are my assumptions influenced by my biases?*," "*have I surrendered to ego?*," "*who am I serving?*", "*am I serving those for whom the interpretation is being done?*" (Romanyshyn 2013).

Reflexive and reflective journaling was an integral part of the interpretive circling activities to help capture my thoughts, feelings and meditations on and of the experiential descriptions of care as they emerged in my consciousness. I used other literary tools such as poetry or drawing to help glean further meanings about the phenomenon (Figures 9.2 and 9.3).

Regular conversations with colleagues were vital in examining, articulating, re-interpreting and reformulating themes and emerging essential themes.

## Thematic contemplations

Consistent with the philosophic framework of hermeneutic phenomenology, coding of data was not used to interpret the meanings of the collected stories. Data coding has quantitative undertones and restricts analysis to reporting on the patterns in the written, black text. Instead, deliberate consideration was given to the shared themes revealed by individual experiences in the black text and, most importantly, in the white spaces: what is not being said but is present in the story. Themes are understood as the "*structures of experience*" or "*the form*

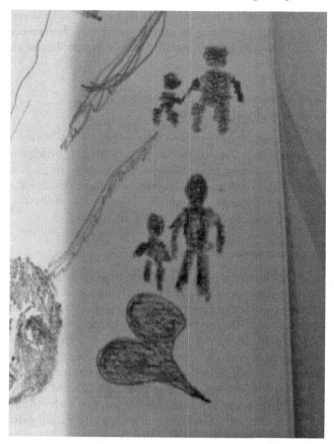

*Figure 9.3* Drawing to Express the Emergent Theme Care Full Mattering

*of capturing the phenomenon one tries to understand*" (van Manen 1990, 79). The meanings given to the phenomenon of care were uncovered through meditations, conversations, daydreaming, journaling and other literary acts (van Manen 1990). Notions uncovered in the interpretations of individual accounts were assigned to the meanings and understandings of the phenomenon of care through "*a very attentive attunement to 'thinking' and listening to how the texts speak*" and the nuances of the phenomenon (Smythe et al. 2008, 1389).

Initial interpretations of the collected stories uncovered provisional themes. These provisional themes remained flexible and changed and/or were reworded as meanings and understandings of the phenomenon unfolded. This unfolding combined intuiting and "*compassionate ways of knowing*" with the academic rigour of human science research (Anderson and Braud 2011, 16). This hermeneutic interpreting continued and evolved into further contemplative writing, attempting to bring to light the essence of everyday reality.

Working with phenomenon was a path of tenacious wondering, thinking, writing and saying out loud what is mostly unspoken. This path led to the emergence of themes of what seemed "to matter." These themes were shaped and re-shaped in the writing, reading, re-writing, re-reading interpretive hermeneutic process. Informed by the writings of Heidegger and Gadamer, powerful ontological themes emerged.

## Working with phenomenon: the dark edges revealed as philosophical notions

In interpreting the lived experiences, a light shines on the "dark edges" of the unseen. In shining a light towards the lived experience of participants, revealed three notions that mattered most: "Care as always mattering"; "Care as play/ play as care" and "Care as being-safe-at-home." It must be noted that while these notions are considered under separate headings, ontologically they must be viewed as parts of the whole of the nature of care-*ing*.

### Care as always mattering

At the heart of HRM rhetoric is the declaration that "People are our most important asset." The appearance of care and concern for people is designed into the policies, procedures and imbued in the governance of relationships at work. The theory and practice of HRM has the guise of care and concern for people first. The ongoing rhetoric creates an expectation that being with and supporting people in organisations matters most. Ontologically, care and concern is always mattering, as we are always beings-in-the-world-together (Heidegger 1992). However, in the telling of the stories, the phenomenon of care in HRM revealed as always mattering either in its presence or absence in encounters with others.

I named the "ishness" of the presence of caring as care full mattering, that is full of care, where relationship and people matter most. The following story reveals care full mattering.

> I worked with a manager who wanted to be respectful and kind and listen to people and that really changed things. People are feeling happier, more appreciated and valued.

I named the "isness" of the absence of caring as care less mattering. That is, encounters with others that revealed a lack of caring and concern for people and relationships. This story reveals care less mattering.

> I don't need HR anymore. They do their job in terms of organising interviews etc. If you had an HR issue, I would worry about sending you over there to get support. Before I'd send anybody to HR that I thought was a bit vulnerable. I'd have to make sure there was somebody there in HR who really knew the policy and was also kind and listening.

As we are always being-in and belonging-together in the world, care is always mattering in its presence (care full) or absence (care less). Most of the stories in this study revealed institutional HRM rhetoric, rules and regulations, policies and procedures imbued with designs of care, do not shape care full encounters that imbue a sense of community and a sense of life into higher education. That is, the absence of care in everyday encounters is taken for granted.

## Care as play/play as care

Encounters such as in this story reveal people getting caught up in the play or game of understanding.

> I emailed a staff member and asked them to do something. They replied (by email) they're not going to do it. I replied, I am telling you to do this because I need this done, I can't do it because I am doing this. Just do it. And she replied, No you tell one of the admin assistants to do it. I replied, No, I am telling you to do it. And this was an email, and we were in an office next to each other.

A core theme of Gadamer's (2013) philosophical hermeneutics is "spiel" or play (also game or drama) as understanding. In regarding *"understanding as the basic posture of human life"* (Taylor and Mootz 2011, 1), Gadamer gives priority to the seriousness of play as a fundamental ontology of our existence. Gadamer (2013) considers play as our very mode of being and belonging in the world. Yet the seriousness of play, as a fundamental ontology of our existence in the world is taken-for-granted.

In the above story, the exchange reveals conflict and division and the disquieting inability of each participant in the game to reach out to understand and respect the other. This lack of understanding to genuinely relate with and or for one another reveals an absence of care as play.

The absence of care is also revealed as creating facades and being disingenuous in the play.

> One Senior Manager looked like a movie star, but it was like he has Aspergers or something. He made a whole lot of crazy decisions. He had a very silly idea about this university. He thought we were going to be a Cambridge or an Oxford or something for god's sake. He said it at least three or four times and I thought what are you on about? You still haven't got to understand what this place is on about.

The nature of the absence of care drives the play towards trivial, meaningless encounters and limited options.

> I have a performance development meeting (PDM) with each staff member once a year. In one performance review I had to deal with a staff member who was underperforming, and we started the lifting performance process. The other staff members were content in their jobs. They all do their job and do their job well. I've probably had the same conversation 5 times with all of them.

The presence of care as play reveals care full action that improvises and brings forth possibilities.

> Each year we have forms that need to be filled out. The forms can be standardized to suit your own staff. The annual performance review is just to formalize things. But mine are all continuous. Reviews are pointless if you just wait for the review time and speak to your staff in a once a year sit down. It just doesn't work. So reviews with my staff are always ongoing, I speak to them often. I speak to most staff virtually every day.

Rather than being subsumed by the play, care as play is embodied as individuals distinguish their "owned self" in the play while attuned to others as individual whole human beings always already beings in-the-world-together.

## Care as being safe at home

Home sweet home. Home is where the hearth is. There is no place like home. Home and or homecoming inspires stories, songs and poetry describing the being-at-home and returning to dwelling or being-at-home as a distinctive sanctuary in which "to be." In this tradition, John Clare's (2019) poem evokes images of home as a place to return to, where we find joy and comfort and a sense of belonging.

> Muse no more what ere ye be
> In fancys pleasure roam
> But sing (by true inspir'd) wi' me
> The pleasure of a home

In contrast, not being-at-home brings a sense of being restive and lost. This sense of homelessness is revealed in this study as people are uncertain, unsettled and do what it takes to survive as they seek a sense of being-safe-at-home. The stories in this study reveal being-safe-at-home as seeking certainty by retreating into offices and firing out emails, "*this was an email and we were in an office next to each other.*" Others hide behind the "whatness" of titles and the certainty in a defined role in a defined hierarchy, "*Just do it.*" Or they comport façades that close out genuine conversation that might open possibilities to different understandings of their own self and others, "*one Senior Manager looked like a movie star.*" Or they seek groundedness in the certainty of letters, "*your job is safe,*" checklists and prescribed scripts of HRM procedure, "*we started the lifting performance process.*"

Academics in the study compared being-at-home in the context of their workplace as "*being like a war zone,*" where "*the power of one's freedom to respond to circumstances (is) beyond their control*" or refer to relationships as "*processes imposed on staff*" or describe the atmosphere as "*toxic.*" I asked, what is mattering? And when managers "*worry about sending people over there (to HR) to get support?*" I asked what is taken-for-granted?

For Heidegger (1966), the journey home is a journey away from the ontic understandings of worldliness and a turning towards existing authentically. The stories in this study reveal a continued captivation with the rhetoric of HRM policies, checklists and governance that promise to keep us safe-at-home. However, ontologically, there is no safety in the home that has lost its meaning, only survival.

## Re-search as care for the soul

Working with phenomenon is searching for what is already there. My approach, therefore, was a *re*-search, looking anew for the constitutive understanding of what it is to be human and being in the world together. I found "*phenomenology speaks as much to the 'soul' as to the 'mind'*" (Smythe 2012, 6). It is soul-full work.

Heidegger's philosophy challenged me to go beyond thinking objectively (the ontic) and return to the hidden, taken-for-granted meaning in the nature of experience (the ontological); to understand the experience of *careing* rather than what care is or ought to do. I penned the nature of my experience as follows.

> Another turn, another ephemeral moment, dark and then light
> A light muted, fleeting. It shines afresh.

The hermeneutic phenomenological philosophy of Heidegger and Gadamer challenged me to search in a way that is free from rules and pre-thought plans. I wrote down my feelings to keep faith in the process. Below is an extract.

> Feelings of uncertainty steal into my gut as I face the bewildering maze.
> Remember, every lock is its key. Have faith ….

In the end, my re-search was simply a matter of being me: letting go of who I thought I should be and what I should do, and, with raised self-awareness, simply being-there in the midst of what is. In the process of understanding the phenomenon of care, I had re-discovered understandings about myself that I had either masked or forgotten. Coming to understand the phenomenon of care and Being in the world also meant coming to a closer understanding of me. That was the hard part.

At times it seemed I was not getting anywhere. Sometimes it felt the answer was in my grasp. I could *feel* its closeness. The more I tried to grasp what I could not "see," the more "stuck" I felt. It was when I stopped looking for answers in various texts and sat down to write, the thesis wrote itself. With faith in the Darkest, I experienced a sense of magical awareness. I experienced "*the gathering of time*" (Collins and Howard 2006, 78). I claimed the work by surrendering to the re-search and being as one within the phenomenon. I let thinking come through contemplation, drawing and writing. I lost myself in the play, intuiting and self-aware, recognising and responding to the resonance of insight. As Heidegger (1962) wrote, "Dasein" is always/already, constitutively "thinking": simply being-there in the midst of what is, where all is melded into an interconnected oneness.

For Marvin and Dory and their search for Nemo, the end of their journey started with new beginnings they never could have imagined nor purposely sought. I also found as I uncovered new understandings of the phenomenon, I uncovered new and profound understandings of myself and my way of being, and I continue to grow and become in the midst of what is.

Just as important as my "findings" was the transformative nature of being-in the research. I always imagined scholarly endeavour was about locking myself away and shutting out the outside world so I could study and focus on the research, sacrificing time with my family and friends to the work. Instead, I found the opposite. Rather than closing out, I experienced an opening up and reaching out to the world around me. As I grew into the research, so did I grow out of the research experience, ever expanding my sense of who I am and how I am in being-in-the-world with others. Hours of contemplation, conversations, drawing, reading, re-reading, writing and re-writing was, and continues to be my home, my hearth, filled with sublime moments of surprises, serendipity and joy when meanings/understandings become something new in the taken-for-granted.

In contemplating the phenomenon of care, I found I was contemplating my existence as "it is". I literally lived the "lived experience" and continue living with renewed attunement to my surroundings. Inspired by my quest for meaning, it became impossible to lock out the world around me. It was important to keep my connection to the outside world, to be ever present. Meaning came to me as "gems" in every encounter, conversations, books (fiction and non-fiction), newspapers stories, movies, walks along the beach that grew and came together as ideas and new understandings in the taken-for-grantedness of everyday. Inspired by philosophers, asking more, expecting less, being open, to just keep swimming in the depths of darkness, working with phenomenon was an ontological journey into the unknown that affirmed my sense of purpose and openness to possibilities of a hope full future.

## Notes

1. In Western philosophy, a priori means knowledge acquired independently of any particular experience, as opposed to a posteriori knowledge derived from experience.
2. Adapted from Heidegger's key idea from *Being and Time* and the Being of the hammer. To simply stare at the hammer, to think about it as a separate "thing," does not reveal anything of the *Being* of the hammer. In this way, the Being of the hammer is disclosed in its utility, its use: it is *with* the workman, in hammering, that the Being of the hammer is revealed. Care*ing* the Being of care, rather than care as a thing.
3. Void – as Berger (2002) identifies the gap, the empty space, the lifeless space between the reality of experience and the promises of the rhetoric.
4. This is also referred to as a preunderstandings or presuppositions interview.
5. Ethics approval for Project 7210 Title: Care in Human Resource Management (HRM) in higher education granted by the Social and Behavioural Research Ethics Committee (SBRCE) Flinders University on 25 May 2016.

# References

Anderson, R., and W. Braud. 2011. *Transforming Self and Others through Research: Transpersonal Research Methods and Skills for the Human Sciences and Humanities*, Suny Series in Transpersonal Human Psychology. Albany, NY: State University of New York Press.

Atkinson, R., and J. Flint, 2004. "Snowball sampling." Edited by M. S. Lewis-Beck, A. Bryman and T. F. Liao, *The SAGE Encyclopedia of Social Science Research Methods*. Thousand Oaks, CA: Sage Publications, Inc.

Berger, J. 2002. *The Shape of a Pocket*. London: Bloomsbury Publishing.

Caelli, K. 2001. "Engaging with phenomenology: is it more of a challenge than it needs to be?" *Qualitative Health Research* 11 (2):273–281.

Clare, J. 2019. "'Home': a poem by John Clare." *Interesting Literature*, 12 February. https://interestingliterature.com/2019/02/09/home-a-poem-by-john-clare/.

Collins, J., and S. Howard. 2006. *Introducing Heidegger*. Edited by R. Appignanesi. Cambridge: Totem Books.

Crowther, S., P. Ironside, D. Spence, and L. Smythe. 2017. "Crafting stories in hermeneutic phenomenology research: a methodological device." *Qualitative Health Research* 27 (6):826–835. doi: 10.1177/1049732316656161

Dick, P. K. 1992. *The Man in the High Castle*. New York: Vintage.

Diekelmann, J. 2005. "The retrieval of method: the method of retrieval." Edited by P. Ironside, *Beyond Method: Philosophical Conversations in Healthcare Research and Scholarship*, Madison, WI: University of Wisconsin Press

Ehrich, L. C. 1999. "Untangling the threads and coils of the web of phenomenology." *Research and Perspectives* 26 (2):19–44.

Finlay, L. 2011. *Phenomenology for Therapists Researching the Lived World*. West Sussex: Wiley-Blackwell.

Finlay, L. 2012. "Debating phenomenological research methods." Edited by N. Frieson, C. Henriksson and T. Saevi, *Hermeneutic Phenomenology Method and Practice*, 17–37. Rotterdam: Sense Publishers.

Gadamer, H.-G. 1998. *The Beginning of Philosophy*. Translated by R. Coltman. New York, NY: Continuum.

Gadamer, H.-G. 2001. *Gadamer in Conversation, Yale Studies in Hermeneutics*. New Haven, CT: Yale University Press.

Gadamer, H.-G. 2013. "Truth and method." Translated by J. Weinsheimer and D. G. Marshall, *Bloomsbury Revelations Series*. London: Bloomsbury Academic. Original edition, 1975.

Gelven, M. 1989. *A Commentary on Heidegger's Being and Time*. Revised ed. DeKalb, IL: Northern Illinois University Press.

Giles, D. 2008. "Exploring the teacher-student relationship in teacher education: a hermeneutic phenomenological inquiry." Doctor of Philosophy, Faculty of Health and Environmental Sciences, Auckland University of Technology.

Giles, D. 2016. "Welcome address." hermeneutic phenomenological research in practice: engaging with lived experiences, 182 Victoria Square Adelaide South Australia, 11 and 12 April.

Heidegger, M. 1962. *Being and Time*. New York, NY: Harper & Row.

Heidegger, M. 1966. *Discourse on Thinking*. Translated by J. M. Anderson and E. H. Freund. New York, NY: Harper & Row.

Heidegger, M. 1968. *What Is Called Thinking?* Translated by F. D. Wieck and J. G. Gray. New York, NY: Harper and Row.

Heidegger, M. 1992. *History of the Concept of Time: Prolegomena/Martin Heidegger.* Translated by T. Kisiel. Bloomington, IN: Indiana University Press.

Jackson, M. 2013. "Politics of storytelling: variations on a theme by Hannah Arendt." http://ebookcentral.proquest.com/lib/flinders/detail.action?docID=3439364

Moules, N., G. McCaffrey, J. C. Field, and C. M. Liang. 2015. "Conducting hermeneutic research: from philosophy to practice." Vol. 19, *Critical Qualitative Research: Critical Issues for Teaching and Learning.* New York, NY: Peter Lang Publishing.

Nixon, J. 2017. "Hans-Georg Gadamer: the hermeneutical imagination." Edited by P. Gibbs, *Springer Briefs in Education.* London: Springer.

Patton, M. Q. 2002. *Qualitative Research and Evaluation Methods.* 3rd ed. Thousand Oaks, CA: Sage Publications, Inc.

Polkinghorne, D. E. 1988. *Narrative Knowing and the Human Sciences, SUNY Series in Philosophy of the Social Sciences.* Albany, NY: State University of New York Press.

Polkinghorne, D. E. 1989. "Phenomenological research methods." Edited by R. S. Valle and S. Halling. In *Existential-Phenomenological Perspectives in Psychology,* Boston, MA: Springer.

Reich, W. T. 1995. "History of care." The University of Georgetown, accessed 15 October. http://care.georgetown.edu/Classic%20Article.html.

Romanyshyn, R. D. 2013. "The wounded researcher: research with the soul in mind." Edited by G. Mogenson, *Studies in Archetypal Psychology Series.* New Orleans, LA: Springer Journal, Inc.

Smythe, E. 2003. "Uncovering the meaning of 'being safe' in practice." *Contemporary Nurse* 14 (2):196–204. doi: 10.5172/conu.14.2.196

Smythe, E. A., P. M. Ironside, S. L. Sims, M. M. Swenson, and D. G. Spence. 2008. "Doing Heideggerian hermeneutic research: a discussion paper." *International Journal of Nursing Studies* 45 (9):1389–1397. doi: 10.1016/j.ijnurstu.2007.09.005

Smythe, L. 2012. "Discerning which qualitative approach fits best." *New Zealand College of Midwives Journal* 46 (June):5–8.

Taylor, G. H., and F. J. Mootz. 2011. "Gadamer and Ricoeur: critical horizons for contemporary hermeneutics." Edited by F. J. Mootz and G. H. Taylor, *Gadamer and Ricoeur: Critical Horizons for Contemporary Hermeneutics,* London: Continuum International Publishing Group.

van Manen, M. 1990. *SUNY Series, The Philosophy of Education: Researching Lived Experience: Human Science for an Action Sensitive Pedagogy.* Albany, NY: State University of New York Press.

# 10 Being an educator as "having-been"

*Joshua Spier*

## Abstract

My doctoral study explored the phenomenon of "being an educator" in higher education, specifically, in the niche field of youth worker education. Using a hermeneutic phenomenological approach, I conducted interview conversations with Australian Youth Work lecturers about their lived experiences of being an educator in the university. I then drew on Heidegger's account of temporality when interpreting these stories, which revealed ontological dynamics that, though integral to a person's everyday experiences of "being" as an educator (including my own), had become concealed from me in the everyday of teaching. Re-seeing what had become hidden enabled me to renew and expand my own pre-understandings of how it "is" to be in the university work-world as an educator.

In this chapter, I focus on just one of Heidegger's notions that captured my thinking, helping to unlock my interpretive analysis of crafted stories and enriched my pre-understandings. Encountering Heidegger's notion of "having-been-ness" enabled me to re-see how, as human beings, having a sense of our own living past is essential to our being as educators in the world. Heidegger's unpacking of ways we exist as "having-been" also illuminated variable ways that educators are always living in relationship to their own having-been-ness. I present examples of participants' stories, accompanied with some interpretive comments, to reveal how an ontological interplay, in relation to an educator's own having-been-ness, is mostly taken-for-granted in the everydayness of teaching and working in the university sector. Overall, I show how engaging with Heidegger's writings on everyday temporality can be useful for the task of interpreting phenomenological data for hidden yet essential ontological aspects of phenomena.

## My situatedness leads me to the phenomenon

My doctoral study (2012–2016) sought to reveal the integral ontological features ("existentials") that constitute the human experience of "being" a Youth Work lecturer in the everyday context of Australian higher education. Voiced another way, my research project was about digging down to the roots of being a Youth Work educator – the existential roots that infuse the work of Youth Work lecturers with meaning and significance (even when those roots are overlooked and forgotten in the busyness of everyday academic work).

My prior experiences as a lecturer for six years within a Youth Work Bachelor degree drew me to this research topic. As a novice lecturer, I looked for and found

DOI: 10.4324/9781003081661-10

an availability of literature to help shape my practice. Written by other more experienced and leading Youth Work lecturers across Australia, this body of literature was very instructive in terms of educational values, curriculum content and pedagogy. I also found well-constructed justifications for why speciality Youth Work degrees matter. For example, Judith Bessant and Michael Emslie (2014) make a strong case for the existence of Youth Work degrees, arguing that bachelor programs like the one in which I was teaching are important because they induct aspiring youth workers into the specialist knowledge, practice and ethical capacities that set Youth Work apart from other approaches to working with young people. Yes, I nodded in agreement when reading this literature – university *Youth Work education matters* (Bessant and Emslie 2014). But this material is more ontic in focus, while my budding concern was to bring awareness to the ontological experiences: What about the people who teach these degrees? What are our experiences? Do they *matter*? Do *we* matter? I noticed that the experience of teaching in these important Youth Work degrees and how this common experience is rendered meaningful for people who are instrumental in providing Youth Work degrees had been overlooked. I was an insider looking at what I had missed rather than a detached outsider looking in. I began by interrogating my assumptions – what did I think made my experiences as a lecturer meaningful? As T. E. Eliot (1963, 194) wrote: "*We had the experience but missed the meaning*".

And what about others outside of my immediate context who also teach in Youth Work degrees? How are our common and contrasting experiences as educators in this niche academic field rendered meaningful for us? How are these experiences meaningful to me? The phenomenon was beckoning.

## How the research design was developed and evolved

Even though, as educators, we may rarely give existential questions like "What does it mean to be an educator?" serious thought, our background sense of what it means to be an educator continuously and implicitly directs our pedagogic involvement in the world of higher education. So, pivotal to my research design was planning to gather the kind of data that would most vividly speak to the heart of the experience itself – data that would not give voice to people's opinions or concepts of what it means, but rather their detailed accounts of their concrete experiences as educators (van Manen 1990; 2014). It became clear to me that in hermeneutic phenomenology, the texts that move closer to the experience itself are people's stories about their experiences of specific events that they have lived through. Clarifying the kind of data I needed drew me forward. But I wondered: how can I gather lecturers' stories? How can I enable them to tell stories that could reveal the hidden existential meanings of being a Youth Work educator?

It was important to be grounded by van Manen et al.'s (2007) caution that sometimes it may appear that a researcher has generated a phenomenological text comprised of people's experiential accounts, but instead, what has really been gathered are the opinions, perceptions, views and explanations voiced by the participants – not accounts of the experiences themselves. It was important that

I was able to recognise the kind of text that I was after – a set of "lived experience stories" (LES) that could let the meaning of my phenomenon show itself *as it is lived*. van Manen's (2014) outline of the narrative structure of an LES[1] was helpful and gave me guidelines to use when gathering narrative material via the interviews, and later, when crafting the raw interview transcripts into exemplary stories of lived experience. An LES (1) is a very short and simple story, (2) usually describes a single incident, (3) begins close to the central moment of the experience, (4) includes important concrete details, (5) often contains several quotes (what was said, done, and so on), (6) closes quickly after the climax or when the incident has passed and (7) often has an effective or "punchy" last line (252). Working with this kind of story has since been further described within the philosophical context of hermeneutic phenomenology (Crowther et al. 2017).

Having come to appreciate the structure of LES, I was then confronted with the challenge of how to gather them from others in a sensitive and ethical manner. Although there are different ways that phenomenological researchers gather their research text, I saw that interviewing was the recommended vehicle through which to elicit participants' lived-experience stories in hermeneutic phenomenological studies (Crowther et al. 2017; Giles 2009; Smythe 2011; Smythe et al. 2008).

Encountering Hans-Georg Gadamer's (2013) and Heidegger's (1962) insights about the conversation were helpful. For them, it is through conversation that what it means to be (including to be human) is disclosed to us (Dahlstrom 2013, 61). I recognised that it is through the unpredictable "play" of conversation that understanding about human experience is mutually accessible for us (Gadamer 2013). At this point, my research design fell into place – I was setting out to gather a set of LES by inviting other Youth Work lecturers – amid the play of interview conversations – to recount their experiences of teaching in undergraduate Youth Work education. As a researcher, this meant entering the "play" as a conversational partner. The Social and Behavioural Research Ethics Committee (SBREC) at Flinders University granted ethics approval for the study on 2 May 2013 (Project number 6012).

The 11 study participants were lecturers from 5 different higher education providers across Australia who had recent experience of lecturing in a Youth Work degree program. The participants all taught Youth Work–specific units[2] or other specific units that were integral to the Youth Work degree like applied sociology, social policy, professional ethics, community development and social research. All participants were involved in curriculum design.

Reflecting after the first two interviews, I realised that the data gathered was theoretical in nature. For example, one participant was keen to talk about the specific values and pedagogy that they thought should underpin university-based Youth Worker education. It became clear that I needed to adjust my approach. It was evident that I needed to be more direct in asking for them to tell stories about their concrete experiences. Friesen (2012), Giles (2009), Smythe (2011) and van Manen (2014) provide guidance in the tact of guiding the conversation away from theory and explanation towards descriptions of experience in terms of personal life stories.

To encourage participants to tell stories about their specific experiences as educators, I asked open-ended questions in ordinary language, for example:

- What do you do as a lecturer?
- Tell me about a time when you felt "this is why I do what I do" (or "this is what it means to be an educator")
- Tell me about a time when you found it difficult to be a lecturer

To invite and contextualise the conversation, my opening question was: How did you come to be teaching in the Youth Work program? While my original purpose was to use this question to open conversation, what surprisingly emerged later in my interpretive analysis was that the rich stories generated by this question (about a person's *prior* experiences) uncovered an integral feature of the experience under investigation, that is, our living past as essential to our experience as an educator.

Occasionally, participants would offer a story of a specific event in condensed form. In these instances, I learnt to invite them to expand on the specific circumstances surrounding this event and what was happening for them as the event was unfolding. This meant using probes like: What were you doing at that time? What does that mean? What happened to you at that moment? Why do you say that? How do you know that? It was important to maintain an interesting disposition throughout the conversation (Roulston 2010). As I grew in confidence as a phenomenological interviewer, I also learnt that I could follow a less sequential pattern in my questioning. I began to draw links across the participant's stories. I started using probes like: Earlier you mentioned [x], can you tell me a little bit more about that? What you said before has got me wondering if/how/what …? As I journeyed through the interview schedule, I found that I became less reliant on ready-made questions (van Manen 2014, 316).

Each interview was transcribed as a verbatim dialogue between the interviewer and participant. My experience of transcribing the audio recordings was a helpful way of staying near the experience. Once each transcript was completed, I crafted discrete LES related to being an educator (see Crowther et al. 2017). All names used by the participants to refer to other people were removed from the transcript and pseudonyms applied. Each transcript generated a set of distinct stories. I merged these stories into a single document that I named the Master Story Book, containing a total of 90 stories. With the crafted stories completed, the next cycle of deepening interpretation started.

## How I "actually did" the interpretive analysis

Having familiarised myself with my set of stories, I sought to further reveal the existential features of the phenomenon. I entered this process by moving to and fro between individual stories and the whole transcript. To begin my encounter with each individual crafted story, I wrote a short description. Once the description was completed for each crafted story, the next move of interpretive analysis began with the following questions: What is the story about? What is the story telling me about the meaning of being a Youth Work lecturer? It was through writing that I was able to immerse myself in wondering about the phenomenon shown in the story. It was in the play of writing that new possibilities began to emerge.

It is important to note that in my preliminary interpretive writings in relation to the crafted stories, I did not yet draw upon Heidegger's ideas from the philosophical literature. The next step involved a re-reading-thinking-writing-dialogue of the entire suite of crafted stories and initial interpretations and consider how these interpretations might be speaking to the meaning of being a lecturer in Youth Work, vis-à-vis., the phenomenon of interest dwelling in the stories.

When the suite of stories had been interpreted to this depth, my early interpretative writings became the basis of hermeneutic conversations with my supervisors prior to beginning the process again with the next participant. During this back-and-forth activity, I opened my interpretive writings to further wondering in relation to the phenomenon. It was through this dialogical process that my pre-understandings were challenged and possible friction points between the stories and my prejudices became an important matter of playful debate.

Following the early stages of interpretive analysis and writing, I stepped into a deeper interpretive phase of intensively drawing on the philosophic literature, particularly the writings of Heidegger. This allowed phenomenological notions and other ideas from the literature to illuminate further possible meanings integral to the phenomenon. I re-read the crafted stories as a whole text and my early interpretative writings. The goal was to uncover integral ontological structures of the phenomenon that appeared to be in play across all the participant's stories.

A set of emerging themes came into view: foundational dimensions of the phenomenon of "being an educator" as experienced in the context of Youth Work education. van Manen (1990) clarifies that the *"essential quality of a theme … [is that we] discover aspects or qualities that make a phenomenon what it is and without which the phenomenon could not be what it is"* (107). In this way, a good theme is one that allows the crafted stories and interpretive accompaniments to bring the researcher and reader in touch with taken-for-granted understandings that, as such, remain silent to us – just beyond words (van Manen 1990, 112). As Smythe et al. (2008) note, the theme is not *"stripped out of the data,"* but rather, the theme is a way to *"show what we see or hear in a text"* (1392).[3]

## Heidegger's notion of "having-been-ness"

One of the integral meanings of "being an educator" emerged in light of Heidegger's (1962) notion of our "living past" or "having-been-ness." Unlike an item of clothing that we can simply discard, our living past is not something we can get rid of any more than we can escape our own death (Heidegger 1988, 265). Regardless of whether we remember or fail to remember some specific detail from our past, our primordial sense of being someone who has been remains intact (Heidegger 1962, 387; 1988, 265).[4]

Heidegger's notion of having-been-ness does not mean that we are somehow bound by what has happened to us in our past lives, but for each of us, as human beings, our own having-been-ness constantly informs our sense of who we are and are able to be (Heidegger 1962, 32–33; 1966, 265). Moreover, as human beings, the very issue of our own having-been can show up differently in different situations as we go about our everyday lives (Leonard 1994, 54). For example, when I go to watch my children perform in a school concert, my sense that I have been a cricketer is not likely to show up for me, or to others who are there, as mattering (unless perhaps there happens to be a cricket-related song). And yet, this aspect of my having-been-ness may indeed be in play, whether explicitly or not, when I go to join my friends for a game of cricket.

According to this insight, the meaning of our own having-been-ness is never set in stone but is constantly coming to meet us in fresh ways (Dahlstrom 2013, 149; Schalow and Denker 2010). Our having-been is, therefore, a "process" that is always in motion (Heidegger 1962, 374). As such, when immersed in everyday activity, the significance of our own having-been-ness might ordinarily be hidden (Harman 2007, 1). But occasionally, a situation may bring our own having-been-ness into view. Further, there may be times when our having-been-ness may appear to emerge as a matter of concern for others. In these kinds of ways, human beings are always open to the interplay of veiling and unveiling of our own lived having-been-ness (Harman 2007, 3).

Engaging with Heidegger's notion of living past revealed different ways that the interplay of a person's having-been-ness is integral to the meaningfulness of being an educator. Here are two examples of having-been-ness in my interpretive analysis.

## Example 1: When educators recognise their prior having-been-ness as mattering

Throughout the interviews, it became apparent that lecturers were drawn to recall certain experiences in their past that deeply mattered to their present lives as educators. Their stories of being a Youth Work lecturer were often traced back to the beginnings prior to becoming an educator. During the interviews, some educators also seemed to experience a moment of recognising that "*what I am*" and "*what I have been*" merge together, as illustrated by Trish's story. Prior to becoming a lecturer, Trish was a youth worker, running a drop-in centre for young people experiencing hardship (Spier 2018, 68). In the following crafted story, Trish recognises the ongoing meaningfulness of this past experience:

> Why I am at university is connected to right at the beginning because I started off in youth work … I was running the youth centre. We would take these young people, mostly who had failed at school. They had been in institutional care by the time I came across them (aged 14 or 15 when I met them). They had either been in children's homes, foster care, detention centres or in the juvenile mental health facilities – lockups basically. They were all brutalised.

A lot of what I was doing with the drop-in centre was the conversations and where you took those, and that depended on the skill of the worker. One of the things I'd always stressed with the young people was, just be honest: if you break something just let us know.

One young woman had been wearing high heel shoes, she stood on a vinyl chair and her heel went through the chair. And she came and said, Look, I'm really sorry, I've just stood on this chair; it's got a hole in it now. And I said, I'm really glad you told me. She hadn't done it deliberately. But you can get things fixed if you know about it.

The youth officer who was working with me was furious that she had damaged the chair and thought that I should have reprimanded her because of the damage. From my point of view, if you want to build an honest relationship, honesty starts with little things. It's how you show that you respect the young people. It's about how you make little steps. If people can see those learning opportunities wherever they are, it means seeing things differently from the people who are around them in coercive environments.

(Spier 2018, 68)

In this story, Trish recalls her past experience of caring for young people in affirming ways (Spier 2018, 69). The story reveals how her past continues to matter ontologically to her being today as an educator. The importance of this event exceeds the confines of measurable, sequential time (Spier 2018, 69).

## Example 2: When an educator's own having-been-ness "comes back" to them

There are times when a lecturer's understanding of their own way of having-been returns to them. In these moments, an educator reclaims a way they have been with others, a way they seek to repeat as they press into their future practice (Spier 2018, 75). In this following crafted story, Sophie reveals how she recovers her own having-been-ness as an educator following its temporary withdrawal.

Nearly two years ago now, my godson committed suicide at 17 [years of age]. I had already finished the semester. The next time I had to stand in front of a class was the next year. I didn't have the emotional energy to put anything into the class, so there were lots of slides, lots of reading off slides. I didn't care. I yelled at someone in the class. I was rude. Students wrote to me and said, you know, Sophie I need help with my essay – and it would be the day before it was due – and I sent them back an email going, well, you might have wanted to start reading three weeks ago … I turned into a monster.

I've always had really good unit evaluations, but for this one semester, I got really terrible unit evaluations from students in that class. I got some really good ones from the students who are very loyal and know me (laugh). And, I know who they are because they were saying Sophie's always blah

blah blah. But from students who I hadn't had before, and there were quite a number of them in that class: she thinks she's the Queen! (laugh). And, it really threw me.

I was really upset, and I talked to lots of my colleagues about it and they just said, oh it's students, you know, blah blah blah. And, I thought, no! While some of it may have been one or two disgruntled students, and unit evaluations are always flawed – but I really took that on. And, I thought, OK, what's happened to make me go from high satisfaction to she's a bitch basically? Because I had such profound grief I felt that I was just very exposed standing in front of the classroom, and I felt that I just wasn't able to give ...

Teaching can be quite intimate – you're opening yourself up. And I just felt that semester that I couldn't do that; that if I opened myself up like that I'd just be crying – I'd just be a bubbling mess. So that was my really big clunky moment – that I thought, OK Sophie, you know how to do this. You know what it is in the past that has made you a good teacher. You know what students love, and what that is, is just bringing your humanness into the classroom.

I always take a lot of myself into the classroom, so we always begin by talking about, how was your week? And, people go, how's your son going? [...] And we all have a big chat and laugh. So, we bring our shared humanity and all our baggage into the classroom and it enables us to talk about complex things – deep things – and it makes for a really rich learning environment. And, yeah – most recently that was my moment that I've thought – yeah!

(Spier 2018, 75–76)

How did Sophie respond when she received negative comments from students? Did she keep "not caring"? Laugh them off? On the contrary, the "terrible" feedback influenced her disposition: *"It really threw me. I was really upset."* Her sense of being thrown moved Sophie to speak with her fellow educators about this issue (Spier 2018, 76). Upon hearing her concern, her colleagues treated it lightly, suggesting any negative feedback said more about the nature of the feedback-givers or to a flawed evaluation process than it did to any real issue on her part requiring attention. However, this interpretation did not satisfy Sophie. Sophie then had a conversation with herself, one that tried to reckon with a turn in her way of being an educator. What emerged for her was a word of resistance to what her colleagues had just said: "*No!*" (Spier 2018, 77). Here, she rejected the option of ignoring the negative feedback. Instead, it moved her back towards a revealed way she had been in the past – a having-been-ness that she resolved to repeat in her future as an educator (Heidegger 1962; Spier 2018). She avails herself to "take on" the terrible feedback and asked a hard question of herself: What's happened to make me go from high satisfaction to "she's a bitch"?

Sophie began to muse back over the preceding semester. As she pondered what had happened to her, an answer to her own question became clear: *Because I had such profound grief I felt that I was just very exposed* standing in front of the classroom, and I felt that I just wasn't able to give … She realised that each week, she had been unable to *bring herself* to tell her students about what was happening in her life, about her grief (Spier 2018, 77). She grasped that she had been unable to give of herself in the way that she *had been* in her past (Spier 2018, 77). She remembered that her own way of having been an educator was to bring her "humanness" into the classroom (Heidegger 1962, 389; Spier 2018, 77). Previously, she began classes by speaking honestly with students about what was happening in her personal and family life. She recognised that tragic circumstances had thrown her. Consequently, as far as she could see, she had been temporarily unable to repeat her prior way of having been an educator. "I just felt that semester that I couldn't do that; that if I opened myself up like that I'd just be crying – I'd just be a bubbling mess."

Coming back to Sophie were echoes of the "chatting" and "laughter" that she had welcomed and enjoyed with her students in past classes (Spier 2018, 77). Here, with the next semester already upon her, her way of having been with her students came back to her, a returning "openness" that had closed while she was coping with the loss of her godson (Heidegger 1962, 373). As her own way of having been with students came back to her, there is an implicit sense that she moved to repeat it, to bring it once again with her into the upcoming semester of teaching:

> I thought, OK Sophie, you know how to do this. You know what it is in the past that has made you a good teacher. You know what students love, and what that is, is just bringing your humanness into the classroom.
>
> (Spier 2018, 75)

Sophie's story seemed to uncover how an experience of coming back to our own having-been-ness is not always easy. Being brought face to face with a way she once was, in the light of how she found herself to be "now," was not a comforting experience. Indeed, for all of us, our current way of being may sometimes emerge as different to a prior way we have been in the world (Heidegger 1962, 373). And yet, such moments can deliver us back to something that is vital for us.

## Reflections on trustworthiness

I heard qualitative researchers speaking about the importance of trustworthiness, which confronted me with the simple question, "Can people (including me) trust the findings of my research? (also refer to Chapter 13 for further insights into trustworthiness)." However, I found multiple criteria against which the trustworthiness of my research could be evaluated, leaving me at times confused about which criteria I could, well, trust. Like Smythe (2019), I felt like trustworthiness was a checkbox that I needed to tick (4). For me, what helped was turning to the voices of experienced hermeneutic phenomenological researchers whose guidance in the process I was already trusting. I heard Smythe wondering, "What would make a phenomenological hermeneutic study untrustworthy?" (4). For her, an untrustworthy study "tells" the reader what the findings were, rather than "showing" the reader in a way that she is "free to think-along-with the researcher" and come to her own interpretations. To establish this kind of trustworthiness, when reading and re-reading the drafts of my analysis chapter, I took up a reflexive stance, asking myself: Am I "telling" or "showing"? Am I inviting the reader to think along with me, to join my play of thinking? When understood in this way, it is not easy to verify if trust has been established with readers. As a novice researcher, I have come to accept that I am still honing the craft of "showing," and, as such, of creating trustworthy research. My final doctoral thesis was not simply "trustworthy" or "untrustworthy." There were moments of both. One examiner of my thesis, an experienced hermeneutic phenomenological researcher, commented that when she was reading some (not all) of my interpretive commentary on the crafted stories, she felt like she was "being told" what she already knew. Yet at other points, she reported experiencing a "resonance" that drew her into thinking, wondering, in a way that allowed the phenomenon to "shine." Her feedback helped me to become a more trustworthy researcher and writer.

For me, the trustworthiness of my hermeneutic study also lies in openness. Trustworthiness came from recognising and holding open my pre-understandings, in a reflexive manner, and allowing them to be challenged, expanded and renewed through my encounters with the stories that the participants had offered, with the philosophical insights I read, and with how other people responded to my emerging ideas as I shared them in conversation, particularly with my wife Christy, colleagues and supervisors. Trustworthiness grew as I learnt to appreciate there will always be more that I have not yet understood. For example, sometimes, when sharing my emerging ideas with my wife, she would bluntly remark, "You've lost me." While at other times, a phenomenological nod would come from her as I shared insights that drew her to see something about her own everyday life (for example, as a mum) that she had missed or taken-for-granted. I tend to agree with Lawrence K. Schmidt: *"in the end, as in all phenomenologies, it must be left to the thoughtful reader to decide on the accuracy of the phenomenological description"* (Schmidt 2006, 66).

## Challenges encountered along the way

The unforeseen challenges that came during this research were numerous and complex. These challenges related to the sustained intensity of the lived experience of the research itself, the constant meditative attunement to my phenomenon, and the process of letting the research process speak and challenge my own historical situatedness and prejudices (Gadamer 2013; Giles 2009).

For me, a core discipline of doing hermeneutic phenomenology was holding the focus of the phenomenon in question throughout my journey, as my relationship with the research text unfolded towards an opening of fresh ontological understandings (Smythe 2011). In the research journey, my question about the meaning of being a Youth Work educator was always nearby. It pervaded my everyday existence. There was nowhere I could go to flee from its address. Whether I was awake or asleep, working on my research project or attending to some other task, thinking-talking about my research data or resting from it, I was continually engaged with my research question in one way or another (Heidegger 2001, 187; 1966). Being on the hermeneutic path called me to "live the question" (Rilke 2014). Yet through doing this kind of research project, I came to appreciate the original meaning of a word that is used frequently by academics in reference to their research: "interest." As Heidegger reminds us, true interest means to be *"in the midst of things, or to be at the centre of a thing and to stay with it"* (1968, 5).

## Concluding reflections

What advice would I now give to a beginning hermeneutic phenomenological researcher who is looking for guidance? When you begin reading Heidegger's *Being and Time* to inform your interpretive data analysis, expect to "not understand." Your early reading of Heidegger will be hard work and frustrating. Know that you are not alone in this experience. Even trained philosophers find his writing "dense, difficult to grasp" and permeated by *"language for which there is no easy translation, and leaves the reader with more questions than answers"* (Smythe and Spence 2019, 1). However, I encourage you to persevere. Trust that, with the required patience, care, attentiveness, humility, and a little help from well-selected guides and companions, your understanding will come (Smythe and Spence 2019). If at all possible, find and recruit a supervisor who has not only read, grasped (not necessarily mastered) and drawn on Heidegger's writings to inform their own doctoral study and interpretive analysis but who also exudes, as a human being, those same qualities you will need to foster – patience, care, attentiveness and humility. I was fortunate to have had one such supervisor, David Giles. I remember some advice David gave me when I was starting to read *Being and Time* early in my interpretive analysis. I had assumed (falsely) that during his doctoral study, he had read the whole of *Being and Time* from cover to cover, deciphering each notion as he went, and that he was expecting me to do the same. Somehow sensing that I was overwhelmed at the prospect of reading Heidegger, David, a keen fisher, suggested that all I needed to do was *"dip in and out"* of Heidegger's text, *"fishing"* for notions that resonated with my data (see Smythe and Spence 2019, 6). When snaring something that does not resonate, he advised me not to dwell on it but to throw my line back in. When catching a notion that *did* resonate, he said it might not make much sense at first. When I first came across Heidegger's notion of "having-been-ness," it jumped out at me. While puzzling, I felt compelled to understand more. For such occasions, David lent me his well-used copy of Hubert L. Dreyfus's (1991) commentary on *Being and Time* to consult, and this book, along with Graham Harman's (2007) *Heidegger explained* and William Blattner's (2006) guide to *Being and Time*, helped me to keep reading and unlock Heidegger's insights. As I came to understand a notion, I would find myself recalling specific crafted stories that exemplified that aspect of human experience Heidegger was illuminating in his writing, and suddenly, I glimpsed an ontological dynamic in play across my data that I had missed – an insight unlikely to have been given if I had not persevered in the struggle to understand Heidegger's writing. As you open yourself to the struggle, I trust similar gifts await you also.

## Notes

1. van Manen calls this kind of narrative an "anecdote" or "lived experience descriptions (LED)," but I prefer "lived experience story," as do Crowther et al. (2017).
2. In Australia, the words "unit," "subject" or "module" normally refer to an academic "course" as it is referred to in North America, while the word "course" typically refers to the entire program of studies required to complete a university degree.
3. As noted by the reviewers of this chapter, the notion of "essential quality" in HP research is not to be confused with some entity or idea that is fixed, final, absolute or universal. Existential understandings of the ontological dimensions of being human are always in some flux, dynamic and emergent.
4. When considering this ontological theme, it is important to remember that our having-been-ness cannot be isolated from the threefold horizon of lived time to which it belongs. Indeed, every moment of our existence is simultaneously orientated to a sense of who we are able to be, who we have been and who we are (Blattner 2006; Heidegger 1962; 1995). It is critical to bear in mind that this dimension is ontologically inseparable from the unified "threefold horizon" of lived time (Heidegger 1995, 145).

## References

Bessant, J., & Emslie, M. (2014). Why university education matters: Youth work and the Australian experience. *Child & Youth Services*, 35(2), 137–151.

Blattner, W. D. (2006). *Heidegger's Being and time: A reader's guide*. London/New York, NY: Continuum.

Crowther, S., Ironside, P., Spence, D., & Smythe, L. (2017). Crafting stories in hermeneutic phenomenology research: A methodological device. *Qualitative Health Research*, 27(6), 826–835.

Dahlstrom, D. O. (2013). *The Heidegger dictionary*. London: Bloomsbury.

Dreyfus, H. L. (1991). *Being-in-the-world: A commentary on Heidegger's Being and time, division I*. London: The MIT Press.

Eliot, T. S. (1963). *Collected poems 1909–1962*. London: Faber and Faber.

Friesen, N. (2012). Experiential evidence: I, we, you. In N. Friesen, C. Henriksson, & T. Saevi (Eds.), *Hermeneutic phenomenology in education: Method and practice* (pp. 39–54). Rotterdam: Sense.

Gadamer, H.-G. (2013). *Truth and method* (J. Weinsheimer & D. G. Marshall, Trans.). London: Bloomsbury Academic. (Original work published 1960).

Giles, D. (2009). Phenomenologically researching the lecturer-student teacher relationship: Some challenges encountered. *Indo-Pacific Journal of Phenomenology*, 9(2), 1–11.

Harman, G. (2007). *Heidegger explained: From phenomenon to thing*. Chicago, IL: Open Court.

Heidegger, M. (1962). *Being and time* (J. Macquarrie & E. Robinson, Trans.). Oxford: Blackwell. (Original work published 1927).

Heidegger, M. (1966). *Discourse on thinking* (J. M. Anderson & E. H. Freund, Trans.). New York, NY: Harper & Row. (Original work published 1959).

Heidegger, M. (1968). *What is called thinking?* New York, NY: Harper & Row. (Original work published 1954).

Heidegger, M. (1988). *The basic problems of phenomenology* (A. Hofstadter, Trans.). Indianapolis IN: Indiana University Press (Original lectures delivered 1927).

Heidegger, M. (1995). *The fundamental concepts of metaphysics: World, finitude, solitude* (W. McNeill & N. Walker, Trans.). Bloomington, IN: Indiana University Press. (Original lectures delivered 1929–30).

Heidegger, M. (2001). *Poetry, language, thought* (A. Hofstadter, Trans.). New York, NY: Harper Perennial Modern Thought. (Original work published 1971).

Leonard, V. W. (1994). A Heideggerian phenomenological perspective on the concept of person. In P. Benner (Ed.), *Interpretive phenomenology: Embodiment, caring and ethics in health and illness* (pp. 43–64). Thousand Oaks, CA: Sage.

Rilke, R. M. (2014). *Letters to a young poet.* London: Penguin books. (Original work published 1929).

Roulston, K. (2010). *Reflective interviewing: A guide to theory and practice.* Thousand Oaks, CA: Sage.

Schalow, F., & Denker, A. (2010). *Historical dictionary of Heidegger's philosophy* (2nd ed.). Lanham, MD: Scarecrow Press.

Schmidt, L. K. (2006). *Understanding hermeneutics.* Stocksfield, England: Acumen.

Smythe, E. (2011). From beginning to end: How to do hermeneutic interpretive phenomenology. In G. Thomson, F. Dykes, & S. Downe (Eds.), *Qualitative research in midwifery and childbirth* (pp. 35–54). London: Routledge.

Smythe, E. (2019). Commentary on: "A critical analysis of articles using a Gadamerian-based research method" (Fleming & Robb). *Nursing Inquiry, 26*(2), https://doi.org/10.1111/nin.12287

Smythe, E. A., Ironside, P. M., Sims, S. L., Swenson, M. M., & Spence, D. G. (2008). Doing Heideggerian hermeneutic research: A discussion paper. *International Journal of Nursing Studies, 45*(9), 1389–1397.

Smythe, E. & Spence, D. (2019). Reading Heidegger. *Nursing Philosophy, 21*(2), https://doi.org/10.1111/nup.12271

Spier, J. (2018). *Heidegger and the lived-experience of being a university educator.* Cham, Switzerland: Palgrave Macmillan.

van Manen, M. (1990). *Researching lived experience: Human science for an action sensitive pedagogy.* Albany, NY: State University of New York Press.

van Manen, M. (2014). *Phenomenology of practice: Meaning-giving methods in phenomenological research and writing.* Walnut Creek, CA: Left Coast Press.

van Manen, M., McClelland, J., & Plihal, J. (2007). Naming student experiences and experiencing student naming. In D. Thiessen & A. Cook-Sather (Eds.), *International handbook of student experience in elementary and secondary school* (pp. 85–98). New York, NY: Springer.

# 11 Straddling paradigms

## A hermeneutic phenomenological exploration of the experience of midwives practising homeopathy

*Jean Duckworth*

## Abstract

In this chapter, I present insights from my Ph.D. study that used a hermeneutic phenomenological framework to explore the experience of midwives who trained as homeopaths. Homeopathy has become a contested discipline with its practitioners often criticised, particularly when practising within the United Kingdom National Health Service (NHS). After a comprehensive analysis of existing literature, in-depth interviews were conducted with seven midwife homeopaths. The midwife homeopaths' narratives were analysed firstly using the concept of metamorphosis before being framed using a Heideggerian lens, which illuminated a process of transformation into "*Being*" authentic practitioners. This chapter explores how hermeneutic phenomenology was enacted using a range of philosophical notions drawn from hermeneutic phenomenological literature. I describe how I spent time with the narratives whilst also continuing reading and allowing my understandings and interpretations to take shape. I explain the importance of reflexivity in my work and how it enabled new and deeper insights into the world as experienced by the participants in my study.

## Background

As the need for a reflexive stance that foregrounds our pre-understandings and situatedness within our topic areas is an essential aspect of hermeneutic phenomenology research – that is where I begin. My interest in understanding why midwives became homeopaths was first piqued when studying homeopathy in the 1990s. I noticed that a significant number of my fellow students were nurses and midwives, and I pondered on why statutorily registered health professionals would want to train in homeopathy. This interest ebbed and flowed over the years, receding as I qualified and started my own practice, and returning as I began lecturing in homeopathy. Like many health professions, professional homeopathy practise requires its practitioners to be reflective and reflexive and through my journaling I remembered some of the stories I heard as a student homeopath. Whilst public interest in and use of homeopathy was increasing at the time, so was the criticism being levelled towards its practitioners, particularly in more orthodox settings. I remember thinking that their path was not easy and felt dismayed and at times angry when they struggled to garner support or attain

DOI: 10.4324/9781003081661-11

recognition for what they were doing. Similarly, I shared their delight when they achieved recognition or were able to influence some aspect of practice.

I was drawn to exploring the experience of midwife homeopaths, first thinking it was solely a professional interest. My diary entries written at the time of writing my Ph.D. proposal, however, revealed how the confluence of my interests and experiences culminated in the development of my study. I wrote of giving birth to my own children:

> Two weeks before I had my daughter I moved from Oxfordshire to York. I knew no-one in York, it felt alien as though I had been transported to another country. I was 24. The night of my daughter's birth my husband was away on business. It was late and I was in bed, in an unfamiliar house, not home yet. My waters broke. I wondered what to do, I had no friends or family nearby. I rang the hospital, they said it was my first baby and to wait to go in when my contractions were every 5 minutes. I said I was on my own, they did not say I should go in; they said to wait till family arrived or call the ambulance when the contractions were closer. I was scared and rang my husband who said he would come home, but it would take a few hours to get to me. Those 3 hours felt more like 24. I felt alone, and in pain, worried about what to expect during the birth. When he got home, we went to the hospital. My contractions were now coming every 3 or 4 minutes. They admitted me and put me straight into a delivery room, where I remained until my baby was born 12 hours later. They came in occasionally to 'do things,' not to be there for me. It was cold and clinical, I felt surrounded by machines. I felt unsupported, as though I was a hindrance to them (the midwives), it seemed to me as though they felt they had better things to do than be with someone that was not 'trying.' Then when they threatened a forceps delivery for mothers who did not try I felt I had let both myself, and my baby down. Even thinking about my birth experience is visceral, and I start to think about how it could be different, to deconstruct it, and replay it with me as I now am, and with my 'ideal' midwives.

Through writing in my journal, I began to realise how important my previous experience was and how it had led me towards my research question. Giving birth had been an important milestone in my life and had punctuated many of the discussions and interactions I had as a woman, mother and as a homeopath. Through the negative experience as a mother giving birth, I developed an image of the "ideal midwife." She, or he, would be technically proficient (that would be a given), but they would also be with me throughout, supporting me, and act as an advocate for the birth I wanted. I had a birth plan, but because it had been developed during my time in Oxfordshire, it was ignored, and I was not confident enough to challenge the midwives attending my labour. I felt that they believed they knew best and I became a passive recipient of their care. This picture of the "ideal" midwife, as competent, caring, supportive and listening stayed with me, like a soundtrack, as I continued to talk to other women and further strengthened by the midwives, I met who wanted to become homeopaths.

Becoming a homeopath, working with pregnant women, and teaching homeopathy added the expectation that homeopathy was useful during pregnancy and childbirth. I had also, by the time I started my study, been the Professional Conduct Director of my registering body, The Society of Homeopaths, for three years and this added yet another layer of beliefs and experiences. Part of this role required that I had to address the issues that arose when individuals are members of different professions. There can be boundary issues and I remained unsure about whether homeopathy could successfully be incorporated into another professional discipline. This question encompassed notions of a professional's scope of practice and whether homeopathy was a medicine that could be used within a healthcare profession or whether it was a discrete professional discipline. As I started to read around the topic, I came to the realisation that the issues were more varied and complex than I had initially determined, and my own views too simplistic.

My doctoral thesis, entitled "*Straddling paradigms: An interpretive hermeneutic exploration of the practise of midwife homeopaths*" Duckworth (2015) told the story of how individuals navigate the space between professions. In this instance, a contested space, as midwifery is framed within the current "normal science" of standard health care provision whilst homeopathy is perceived to stand in opposition to these health care norms.

## How a literature review "fits" into the research design

Unusually, and perhaps counter-intuitively for a phenomenological study, I conducted a mixed method systematised review of the literature at the start of my study. This was, in part, a recommendation from my supervisory team, who suggested a systematised approach to reviewing the literature as a way of ensuring that I could identify any gaps in what is known on the topic. This is key when completing a Ph.D. as it requires an original contribution to knowledge, and so a review is a means of eliciting what is already known. In choosing to start with a review, I considered the ongoing debate about the best time to review the literature. Holloway and Wheeler (2010) cite earlier researchers such as Glaser (2004), who reason that reviewing the literature too early in a project is inadvisable as it could directly influence the later empirical research. However, this could be a conceit as without any preconceptions there are no questions. Holloway and Wheeler (2010) make the argument that often researchers come to research with prior knowledge, as in my own case, and therefore pre-conceptions will always exist. Smythe and Spence (2012, 16) agree and add that when undertaking a review of the literature for a hermeneutic study, the reviewer stands "*at the crossroads of all their fore-understanding.*" This means that in coming to the literature, I already had a starting place or understanding of the topic, described by Heidegger as my "fore-having," which arises out of my "drawnness" towards the contested space between midwifery and homeopathy. In addition to this, I also possessed Heidegger's notions of "fore-sight" and "fore-conception."[1]

This "fore-sight" revealed itself in my having an understanding about which search terms I might choose, which journals were likely to include relevant studies and "fore-conception" where I already had a sense about what I might find in the literature. My mind had been occupied for many hours thinking about the study, how it might play out, what I would find. For Smythe and Spence (2012, 16) this *"fore-conception"* is the *"most dangerous aspect of understanding."* As I had come to the study with some knowledge about the topic, and I have to admit, a bias built on many years of being a mother, homeopath and educator, I had to consciously remain open to the possibility, or in retrospect, would say likelihood, of my "fore-conception" being challenged by my reading and findings. This notion of remaining open to the challenge was one revisited at every stage of my study.

For Smythe and Spence (2012, 16), a literature review is also the opportunity to move between my *"already-there"* understandings and those *"that may be seen or unseen in the text"* and allowed me as the researcher to grow my understanding. By conducting a substantive literature review at the start, I placed myself in a position to engage in a continuous process of remaining alert to emerging literature, which I regularly revisited to ensure that no relevant literature had been missed.[2] The literature review, in conjunction with my reflexive work to understand my stance, enabled me to explore literatures about the efficacy and effectiveness of homeopathy in maternity care and the attitudes towards and use of homeopathy in U.K. maternity care. Both parts of the review were important in understanding more about the contested nature of homeopathy within midwifery care.

Prior to conducting the literature review, my pre-conceived ideas and fore conceptions led me to thinking that my study could reveal stories about power imbalances (Foucault 2019), or the barriers and facilitators of homeopathy practise within a biomedical system. This was a time of questioning and thinking, and my diary was used to write down my thoughts which in turn enabled me to critically reflect as I moved through various levels of understanding. At times I felt that I understood where I was yet to go, but at other times felt woefully at sea with little understanding. Although I have said that I thought my study might include Foucauldian notions around power, I felt and still feel a resonance with phenomenology. I had already become attuned to phenomenology as a student of philosophy and as a homeopathic practitioner working with the lived experiences of patients. I explored other methodologies, and whilst I could have used them, none of them gave me the "feeling" of being quite as "good a fit." It was the alignment of the question and my experience that kept drawing me towards hermeneutic phenomenology as the best way to explore the phenomenon.

## How the research design unfolded

Initially, I intended to recruit participants via the midwifery and homeopathy public registers. This brought its own issues as none of the registers provided details of ancillary qualifications. So, neither register held records of other professional qualifications. To resolve this, I used purposeful sampling, first turning to the midwife homeopaths I trained alongside or who had previously been my students. I then used a snowballing approach and asked my participants if they knew of any other midwife homeopaths. After I had exhausted this avenue, I used the internet to search for independent midwives who used homeopathy as well as asking the Independent Midwives organisation. Eventually, I found seven midwife homeopaths who expressed an interest in being interviewed.

Of the seven UK midwives who agreed to meet with me, two (Zoe and Emily) practised midwifery in the UK National Health Service [NHS] and homeopathy in non-NHS settings, three (Chloe, Grace and Jessica) were no longer practising as NHS midwives but practised homeopathy in non-NHS settings, and Gina combined midwifery and homeopathy but as an independent midwife. One (Tina) withdrew from the study, however, was practising both midwifery and homeopathy in an NHS setting at the time of my study. Tina made a decision to withdraw after she had been interviewed as she felt that her openness might lead to her being recognised due to so few midwives practising homeopathy in the NHS at the time.

I had originally envisaged interviewing ten participants and was disappointed when I only recruited six. I wrote in my diary, "How many is enough?," expressing my frustration at not being able to reach participants to tell me their experience. To seek reassurance, I turned back to my earlier reading about sampling in phenomenological studies. Cresswell (2013) reported phenomenological studies where the number of participants had been as low as one (Dukes 1984) and as many as 325 (Polkinghorne 1989). Cresswell (2013, 5) wrote that in a phenomenological study, *"long interviews with up to ten people"* are optimal. Englander (2012) suggested no less than three, whilst Dukes (1984) recommended between three and ten participants. Giorgi (2009) believes, however, that it is the depth and quality of the data obtained that is important, not simply the number of interviews undertaken. Englander (2012), in discussing sample size, states that the phenomenological researcher seeks to explore the experience of the phenomenon, not how many people have experienced it. Likewise, Smythe (2011) suggests the quantity of interviews is not the focus, data gathering in this genre of research is more focused on having "sufficient data" that reveals the phenomenon of interest. I was reminded that as a phenomenological researcher I was not attempting to address issues surrounding generalisability or representativeness, or saturation.

The tension resolved itself as my interviews progressed and there was a point where I felt that I had collected enough data for my study and that I would be able to provide an interpretation that was both convincing and transparent.

By conducting unstructured interviews, I aimed to explore how the phenomena of "being a midwife homeopath" were perceived and experienced. I wanted to gather deep, comprehensive, and textured information and perceptions, and using unstructured interviews enabled me to understand each participant's experience and the meaning they ascribed to it (Seidman 2012). Whilst often the participant is given the choice of interview location for a face-to-face interview because many of them lived and worked across the country, I offered the alternative of telephone or Skype interviews. Five participants chose a telephone interview because it provided them a greater degree of freedom in choosing convenient days/times.

Whilst it is not the most common method, telephone interviews have been and continue to be used in phenomenological research (Drabble, Trocki, Salcedo, Walker and Korcha 2016).

I paid careful attention to several concerns expressed about telephone interviews, including that in addition to the potential lack or rapport and empathy, there may be a loss of contextual and non-verbal data (Novick 2008). Novick believes there is considerable bias against the use of telephone interviews, and they are seen as being a much less desirable method than face-to-face interviews. However, he suggests that telephone interviews offer benefits in allowing a participant to feel relaxed and more able to disclose personal or sensitive data. He argues that there is no evidence that would support the hypothesis that telephone interviews inhibit the collection of quality data. Sweet (2002) conducted a phenomenological study with nurses and found telephone interviews to be both methodologically and economically valid stating that qualitative researchers should not solely rely on face-to-face interviews. I found no discernible difference in the depth or quality of the data from the telephone interviews when compared to those collected via face-to-face interviews. At the time, I wrote in my reflexive diary:

> I did my second interview today, it was by phone, and I really enjoyed listening to 'x.' I was worried that there may be something 'missing' from the interview, that by not being there with them that we may not connect, and they may choose not to tell me the full extent of their experience. I was pleased that this doesn't seem to be true, and 'x' was open, and honest.

In a world increasingly global in focus and currently gripped by a COVID-19 pandemic, many qualitative researchers have needed to move to online interviewing (e.g. Zoom, Skype, Microsoft Teams and telephones) – my own experience is that such approaches do not provide barriers to conducting fruitful phenomenological research.

## Undertaking the analysis

The six interviews generated a significant quantity of data and notes for analysis. Initially, I was tempted to use software such as NVivo or MAXQDA to help with the analysis. I thought this would help to speed up my data handling and make it easier to organise and explore the data. I am technically competent and teach online courses, so I was not fearful about using technology. Instead, there was a drawness to listening and transcribing. It was by living with the stories, reading and re-reading them and reading philosophical texts that my own insights began to occur. Some things quickly became apparent, yet others remained hidden from view. Gadamer (1975) calls this the space where we are free to "play" so that understanding and interpretation can be reached. For Heidegger, understanding and interpretation are equiprimordial constituents of *Daesin*. In the process of reaching an understanding, we interpret or work out the possibilities projected

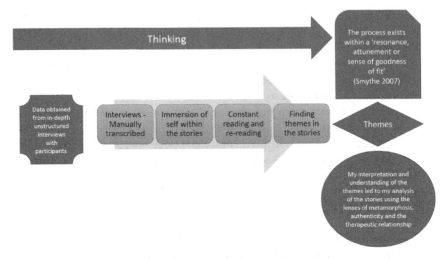

*Figure 11.1* Analysis of Data

in this understanding (Heidegger 1962). Kirby and Graham (2016, 9) write that for Gadamer, "play" *"discloses the full context of any given situation by promoting a freedom of possibilities within the horizon of one's own life world (the world directly and immediately experienced)."* This "play" is dynamic and privileges emergent understandings. Dunne (1993) calls the thing that allows "things to be revealed" as "thinking." It is "thinking" that allows things to be revealed, not by *"working out"* but instead, it happens through a "letting come." For me, the process of *"letting come"* involved an iterative, interpretive process that continued for months. This "thinking" was not to be hurried as my thoughts matured and understandings developed.

The midwives' stories were viewed separately and gathered so both their individual and collective experiences could be understood. I "played" with the data allowing patterns to reveal themselves and generated theme statements to capture the meaning inherent in the data. To make sure that I was at ease with my interpretation of my participants' story/stories, I spent time re-listening the interviews whilst continuing to reflect. Following the principles in Gadamer's hermeneutic circle, it is not possible to examine each story independently from the meaning of the whole text or the whole text without reference to each story. There is a mutual dependence: individual text elements change their meaning following the whole and the whole changes with its parts. The hermeneutic circle is open and transparent circle and allows concepts to flex and change with time (Dobrosavljev 2002). Figure 11.1 shows how I analysed my data.

It was after reading and re-reading, or "thinking" about their stories using a hermeneutic phenomenological approach that the ideas of a personal and professional transformation became apparent to me. Initially, my thoughts were of the midwives following a journey, and whilst I could see that in their stories, I realised that something else was happening. Their stories were not about

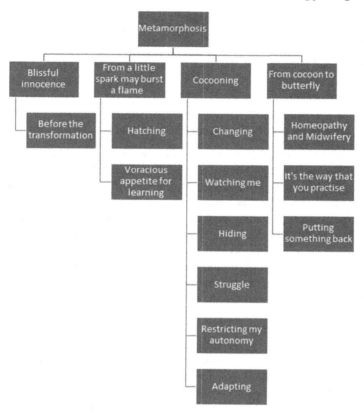

*Figure 11.2* Themes

someone simply learning a new technique, process or procedure. Instead, it was about them inhabiting a new paradigm of thinking which in turn affected their identity. The midwife homeopaths had fundamentally changed and transformed through their learning of homeopathy, and this had a direct impact on their midwifery and homeopathy careers. Consequently, the story I presented was one of the midwives' "metamorphosis," and this was used as the overarching metaphor to represent the midwives' experiences. A caterpillar to butterfly metamorphosis represented to me the radical nature of the life changes sustained by the midwife homeopaths as they travelled through this period in their lives. Figure 11.2 shows the themes created.

As shown in Figure 11.2, the analysis process involved the creation of four main themes, Blissful innocence, From a little spark may burst a flame, Cocooning, and From cocoon to butterfly. An outline of each theme is presented as follows:

### Blissful innocence

This theme described the experiences of five of the midwives before they became fully aware of homeopathy (the sixth participant started her journey as a homeopath before becoming a midwife). Jessica told me how she saw midwifery as a "*vocation*" and a place where you "*longed to go everyday … Everybody just helped each other out and always the women were there at the centre, and the women and their babies and families were always at the forefront of our practice.*" I interpreted this "blissful innocence" metaphorically as the first stage of their metamorphosis from egg to butterfly.

### From a little spark may burst a flame

This theme represents the larval stage of metamorphosis to illuminate how the midwives became aware of homeopathy as a possibility. They each experienced a family health issue which in turn led to an "epiphany," a pivotal point where they wanted to learn more about homeopathy. The prompts towards homeopathy came from family, friends and colleagues. In Chloe's case, it was a colleague who suggested it. At the time of the suggestion, she was unaware of homeopathy and what it might offer to her. Grace decided on homeopathic treatment for her daughter, even though she knew very little about it at the time. It was not a rational decision, she said, but a choice she made because she felt she had very few options open to her within the conventional model on offer. She describes how she,

> thought I can't do this to my child so at this point she had started school and I decided, I just said to my husband at the time, I am going to find a homeopath, not really knowing what it was about, not knowing anything about anything really and just thought it is an alternative medicine.

This interest led to the midwives making a momentous decision by embarking on professional training as homeopaths. This I termed "hatching." Jessica and Emily described the moment when they knew what they wanted to become homeopaths. Emily called it a "light bulb moment" whereas Jessica describes how the decision just came "out of the blue one day." For others, it was a more gradual realisation. Zoe described how:

> I had been to college one Sunday and I came back and something clicked during that day, and I just thought 'you know what I am going to leave [midwifery] and obviously we needed the income and all the rest of it and I just thought 'No! I am going to go' and went home and discussed it with my husband who was very supportive, and just said do what you have to.

The midwives became highly motivated students with a "*voracious appetite*" for learning. Chloe describes how she was "*blown away with the philosophy of it all*," whilst Grace reported how "*the more I got to know … the more I wanted to know*".

### Cocooning

I termed the metaphorical chrysalis stage "cocooning" to tell of the midwives' experiences when attempting to transfer their learning into practice. Whilst cocooned insects are rapidly changing, this is not always outwardly apparent. Emily found that "*the whole way I look at life as a person, as a midwife, has changed through homeopathy,*" and Grace reflected on how "*her values changed as a result.*" Cocooning is also a time when insects are vulnerable to attack. Interestingly, the midwives found their traditional environment to be alien and unfriendly towards them during this period. Chloe described how she found it difficult, "*the more I learned about the philosophy, the more I hated my job.*" Some participants found it increasingly difficult to continue to fit in. Jessica recounted how she felt

> Frustrated … I wouldn't' want to …. look after women and give them conventional treatment, drugs, things like that when I know how much better it could be for them using homeopathy, and then I just wouldn't be able to use that at all' and 'I wouldn't want to be dishing out pethidine to people when I can see a far better way forward.

Grace said how she "*was viewed as an oddball, because [she] was going against the grain …. practising homeopathy*" and "*felt there was a bit of witch hunt going on*" and "*had to watch (her) back.*"

### From cocoon to a butterfly

In the final stage, "*from cocoon to a butterfly*" I depicted the eventual emergence of the butterfly. Each participant had changed fundamentally during their training, and this was reflected in choices they subsequently made. All set up private homeopathy practices. In addition, one midwife chose to work as an independent midwife, and a further two as midwives employed by the NHS, one within a practice that offered homeopathy and another who was able to adapt practice to accommodate her beliefs. Neither Zoe nor Emily was prepared to leave midwifery. Zoe said that she continued practicing midwifery as she believed her homeopathy experience gave her something unique to contribute and she could advocate for the mother and family, whilst Emily believed that caring for mothers and their families in a "*holistic way*" was important. What is important is not what choice they made, but that through their exposure to homeopathy, something fundamental changed for each of them and this change resulted in them having to make some resolute choices.

To further develop my understanding of the stories, I used a technique called "freewriting." Freewriting is when the writer tries to write for a predetermined length of time, up to 20 minutes, without a break or considering grammar or style of writing. It allows for a free flow of ideas and helps develop writing skills. Prior to freewriting, my writing was overly structured; I started at the beginning and tried to get every paragraph "right" before moving onto the next, eventually reaching a conclusion. This was both time-consuming but also very restrictive. I felt that my version of "freewriting" in my journal unshackled me from doing this, and it not only increased the flow of my ideas but also removed the filter from my thoughts (see Goldberg (2005) *Writing Down the Bones*). Being unshackled, I was able to write whatever came to mind as a type of reflection. Derrida (cited in Van Manen 2006) wrote that

> writing creates a space that belongs to the unsayable. It is in this writerly space where there reigns the ultimate incomprehensibility of things, the unfathomable infiniteness of their being, the uncanny rumble of existence itself, but in this fleeting gaze, we also sense the fragility of our own existence, of our own death, that belongs to us more essentially than anything. (718)

Through my freewriting, I started to re-engage with my earlier readings of Heidegger. This felt like "coming home," and I began to see how the participants' stories were reflected in his writings. Significantly, I became aware of how often I was perceiving the notion of "authenticity." It is worth noting that Heidegger's writings on authenticity have been the subject of broad discussion (Sherman 2009; McManus 2019; Varga 2001), and here I do not intend to repeat those but to explicate my own understanding of "authenticity," and share my interpretation of its relevance to the midwives' stories.

As I think about writing this chapter, I become aware of the passage of time and am mindful that my reading, thinking and understanding about authenticity has expanded and matured in the decade or so since my original study. Consequently, although much of what I write here is rooted in the original study, this reflexive account of it has been updated to include elements of my subsequent reading and thinking.

## Authenticity

The nature of authenticity is a major theme for Heidegger, and to understand it, it is necessary to explore it within the context of his philosophy of "Being." Heidegger concerned himself with the ontological question of "Being," which he called *Dasein*, translated from the German "Being there" or "Existence."

As Dasein, we experience "Being-in-the-world," in that we as human beings are embedded and inseparable from our lifeworld (Horrigan-Kelly, Millar and Dowling 2016). We are *"thrown"* into the world as a *"a product of [our] time, place and culture"* (Sherman 2009, 1). It is Dasein's nature to become absorbed in the rhythm of our everyday lives, and Heidegger calls this tendency the "they" or "Das Mann." When acting in this mode we tend to think and act as others do and in the everydayness of our existence, we have a tendency to forget ourselves and thus surrender our uniqueness. Heidegger states that in our everydayness, we can experience "tranquility" and can be deceived that everything is well, when it is not (Heidegger 1962, 231). This engagement with the "they" world should not be perceived as derogatory; instead, for Heidegger, this mode of being, which he named as "inauthenticity," is a fundamental state of being. However, Heidegger also considered that as Dasein is capable of understanding, the individual is able to transcend the thrown condition of inauthenticity to experience moments of authenticity (Polt 2013). This can happen when we experience a "mood," in this case, "anxiety" and the world previously recognised by Dasein falls away. Authenticity relates to Dasein having the *"freedom of choosing itself and taking hold of itself"* (Magrini 2006, 232). Anxiety is a constant threat to Dasein's everyday lostness in the "they," although we are very good at turning away from it. It begs the question about what we are turning away from, and for Heidegger, this is always "Being-towards-death." For Heidegger, authenticity is fundamentally related to the relationship of Dasein to death. Heidegger considered that we tend to live our lives, avoiding thinking about death and the finite nature of our existence. He believed that we tend to push the time and nature of our death to the back of our minds, where we can ignore it by retreating into our everydayness. However, when we think about and "own" our own possibility of dying, the everyday world retreats and in this moment of "anxiety," we are alone. This "ownedness" enables a shift in our attention, where Dasein *"authentically understands itself and acts in the world accordingly"* (Sherman 2009). It is a state where we realise our finiteness and can focus on what is important – to take a stand on our existence as something that matters.

## The midwives stories

What follows is my interpretation of the midwives' stories through the lens of Heidegger's notions of inauthenticity and authenticity. Despite homeopathy being historically available in the NHS, choosing to become a midwife homeopath brings with it its own set of challenges. This is largely owing to the contested nature of the discipline, which leads to a lack of institutional support and ridicule being levelled at its practitioners (Goldacre 2007).

As Dasein, the midwives are "thrown" into a distinct world, bounded by time, place and culture. This inevitably has an effect on the midwives "Being-in-the-world," and they are caught up in inauthenticity in the everydayness of their "run of the mill" personal and working lives. In this state, Heidegger says there is "tranquility." This tranquility, it is argued, can be illusory, and this may have been so for the participants. Before discovering homeopathy, the midwives claimed they were content in their lives and felt a sense of belonging as midwives. The midwives, in their interviews, said how much they had *"loved"* being midwives in the past.

However, what I heard within the narratives was that once the midwives had recognised the tension (anxiety) in their lives they had a choice whether to remain caught up in the "they" or they could choose authenticity. The participants in the study experienced this "tension" when trying to manage family illness, for Chloe, it was when her doctor wanted to prescribe steroid inhalers for asthma, whilst for Emily, the challenge was experienced when she took her baby to the General Practitioner (GP) with an ear infection to be told that babies of three months *"don't get ear infections."* Similarly, Grace, who had a poorly child, states that she just

> thought I can't do this to my child … I just said to my husband at the time, I am going to find a homeopath, not really knowing what it was about, now knowing anything about anything really and just thought it is an alternative medicine.

By choosing to become homeopaths, they were starting to think for themselves and to "*either truly come to grips with (their own) deepest possibility of being, or draw (their) ambitions and self-understanding from what the public says*" (Harman 2006, 60). Their authentic existence came to fruition when the midwives "*owned a standpoint.*" McManus (2018, 1183) provides an example of this as when we appropriate a "*particular vocation or life-project*" or the "*owning of a narrative or life-story.*"

For Grace, the

> final, final, final nail in the coffin came when .... In a home of a first time mum and she was breastfeeding ... I was giving the spiel and showing her what to do, and whilst I was talking I had a very, very powerful vision and I knew then at that point that I would go.

As previously stated, any discussion of authenticity needs to consider "Being-towards-death." For much of the time, we ignore "death" knowing that it will happen, but in some undetermined date in the future, and we live our lives with the infinite possibility that brings (Sherman 2009). Heidegger tells us that, in general, we "flee" from this awareness. It is only when we make a resolute choice, knowing what is valuable and important to us that we can be authentic. When we are no longer evading ourselves, we become "*free for one's own death*" (Heidegger 1962, 307/262). The midwives now have an "ownedness" and as Jessica states, she "*wouldn't go back, I couldn't ... that would not be a possibility at all.*" According to McManus (2018, 267), death is the "*fact that there will be a determinate body of fact about who I will have been, a body the final make-up of which can be determined at any time.*" Therefore for the midwives in my study, through personal circumstance and an associated mood of anxiety, they made a resolute stance for homeopathy to be within the "make-up" of their existence.

## Reflections on the use of hermeneutic phenomenology

In this final section, I offer some of my personal reflections about engaging with this methodological approach. Hermeneutic phenomenology, instead of being driven by prescribed methodological stages, is the adoption of and acting in accordance with an ontological attitude that enables the researcher to retain an open questioning stance (Barak 2020; Crowther, Ironside, Spence and Smythe 2017).

In practical terms, this meant that I engaged in a dialogue with the midwife homeopaths in my study, encouraging them to tell me about their experiences. I remained open to what they wanted to tell me, and these stories were subsequently crafted into powerful shared stories revealing the experiences of midwives transforming into homeopaths. Within phenomenological research, the process of interpretation is a subjective one, with the process bringing about what Gadamer refers to as a "fusion of horizons" (1975) between the stories and researcher. I also employed "epistemological reflexivity" (Dowling 2006), where I reflected upon my theoretical assumptions and perspectives.

It was important for me that when starting this study that I engaged in "thinking" about who I was, why I felt drawn to this study, what my aim for the study was. My own background and the context for the study were written into my early chapters so that I was transparent, and readers could see how I came to the study and what understandings and assumptions (and biases) I already possessed. This reflexivity was continued and written about throughout to enable readers to see my evolving understandings. I contend that the question of who I am is indivisible from the research, but that through reflexivity, I remained open to challenge and to see new possibilities. It is the purpose of hermeneutic phenomenological research to show the reader the stories and invite them to think. It is the reader who will determine if the study is believable (Koch 1996).

The joy for me is that hermeneutic phenomenology aligns with my values and experience, it both enabled and continue to enable me to go beyond the surface, to understand and interpret what lies beneath, and to give a voice to people. It is a real privilege to be part of these phenomenological conversations.

For anyone embarking on a phenomenological study, it is essential is to carry on reading and thinking throughout your study and trust that the phenomenon will reveal itself. I never knew when I would have those "lightbulb" moments of real insight into the meaning, and these could only happen by keeping an open mind. My advice is to ensure that everything is written down in a diary, carry it with you in your bag, pocket, by your bed, the second is to have a really good critical friend that will support you during the tough times and celebrate your successes with you. I would like to acknowledge Dr. Hazel Partington for being that friend.

## Notes

1. The elements mentioned in this paragraph comprise Heidegger's forestructures of understanding.
2. Some Hermeneutic phenomenologists chose to omit a formal literature review, although this can pose a risk when submitting work for postgraduate examinations. Others have conducted a hermeneutic literature review process as part of their theses and dissertations. For an example of this approach, see Crowther, Susan, Elizabeth Smythe, and Deb Spence. (2014). The Joy at Birth: An Interpretive Hermeneutic Literature Review. Midwifery. 30(4): e15.

## References

Barak, A. (2020). Fusing Horizons in Qualitative Research: Gadamer and Cultural Resonances. Qualitative Research in Psychology. DOI: 10.1080/14780887.2020.1854403

Cresswell, J.W. (2013). Qualitative Inquiry and Research Design: Choosing among Five Approaches. London: Sage.

Crowther, S., Ironside, P., Spence, D. & Smythe, L. (2017). Crafting Stories in Hermeneutic Phenomenology Research: A Methodological Device. Qualitative Health Research. 27(6), 826–835.

Dobrosavljev, D. (2002). Gadamer's Hermeneutics as Practical Philosophy. Philosophy, Sociology and Psychology. 2(9): 605–618.

Dowling, M. (2006). Approaches to Reflexivity in Qualitative Research. Nurse Researcher. 13(3): 7–21. DOI: 10.7748/nr2006.04.13.3.7.c5975

Drabble, L., Trocki, K.F., Salcedo, B., Walker, P.C. & Korcha, R.A. (2016). Conducting Qualitative Interviews by Telephone: Lessons Learned from a Study of Alcohol Use among Sexual Minority and Heterosexual Women. Qualitative Social Work. 15(1): 118–133.

Duckworth, J. (2015). Straddling Paradigms: An Interpretive Hermeneutic Exploration of the Experience of Midwives Practising Homeopathy. Available at: http://clok.uclan.ac.uk/12130/

Dukes, S. (1984). Phenomenological Methodology in the Human Sciences. Journal of Religion and Health. 23: 197–203.

Dunne, J. (1993). Back to the Rough Ground: Practical Judgement and the Lure of Technique. Notre Dame, IN: University of Notre Dame Press.

Englander, M. (2012). The Interview: Data Collection in Descriptive Phenomenological Human Scientific Research. Journal of Phenomenological Psychology. 43: 13–35.

Foucault, M. (2019). Power: The Essential Works of Michel Foucault 1954–1984 (Essential Works of Foucault 3). New York: Penguin.

Gadamer, H.G. (1975). Truth and Method. Chippenham: Continuum Books.

Giorgi, A. (2009). The Descriptive Phenomenological Method in Psychology: A Modified Husserlian Approach. Pittsburgh, PA: Duquesne University Press.

Glaser, B.G. (2004). Remodeling Ground Theory. Qualitative Social Research. 5(2): Art 4. Available at: http://www.qualitativeresearch.net/index.php/fqs/article/view/607/1315#g34. Accessed 30 June 2021.

Goldacre, B. (2007). The End of Homeopathy? Available at: http://www.badscience.net/2007/11/a-kind-of-magic/. Accessed 30 June 2021.

Goldberg, N. (2005). Writing Down the Bones: Freeing the Writer Within. Boulder, CO: Shambhala.

Harman, G. (2006). Heidegger Explained: From Phenomenon to Thing. Chicago, IL: Open Court Publishing Company.

Heidegger, M. (1962). Being and Time (trans. J. Macquarrie & E. Robinson). New York: Harper Collins.

Holloway, I. & Wheeler, S. (2010). Qualitative Research in Nursing and Healthcare. 3rd ed. London: Wiley-Blackwell.

Horrigan-Kelly, M., Millar, M. and Dowling, M. (2016). Understanding the Key Tenets of Heidegger's Philosophy for Interpretive Phenomenological Research. International Journal of Qualitative Methods. 1–8. DOI: 10.1177/1609406916680634

Kirby, C. & Graham, B. (2016). Gadamer and the Importance of Play in Philosophical Enquiry. Reason Papers. 38(1): 8–20.

Koch, T. (1996). Implementation of a Hermeneutic Inquiry in Nursing: Philosophy, Rigour and Representation. Journal of Advanced Nursing. 24(1): 174–184. DOI: 10.1046/j.1365-2648.1996.17224.x

Magrini, J. (2006). Anxiety "in Heidegger's Being and Time: The Harbinger of Authenticity" (2006). Philosophy Scholarship. Paper 15. http://dc.cod.edu/philosophypub/1

McManus, D. (2018). Phenomenology, Logic, and Liberation from Grammar. In Wittgenstein and Phenomenology, 47–70. Abingdon: Routledge.

McManus, D. (2019). On a Judgment of One's Own: Heideggerian Authenticity, Standpoints, and All Things Considered. Mind. 128(512): 1181–1204.

Novick, G. (2008). Is There a Bias against Telephone Interviews in Qualitative Research? Research in Nursing and Health. 31: 391–398.

Polkinghorne, D.E. (1989). Narrative Knowing and Human Sciences. New York: State University of New York Press.

Polt, R. (2013). Heidegger: An Introduction. Ithaca, NY, Cornell University Press.

Seidman, I. (2012). Interviewing as Qualitative Research: A Guide for Researchers in Education and the Social Sciences. New York: Teachers College Press.

Sherman, G. (2009). Martin Heidegger's Concept of Authenticity: A Philosophical Contribution to Student Affairs Theory. Journal of College and Character. 10(7). https://doi.org/10.2202/1940-1639.1440

Smythe, E. (2011). From Beginning to End: How to do Hermeneutic Interpretive Phenomenology. In Qualitative Research in Midwifery and Childbirth: Phenomenological Approaches, edited by G. Thomson, F. Dykes & S. Downe, 35–54. London: Routledge.

Smythe, E. & Spence, D. (2012). Re-Viewing Literature in Hermeneutic Research. International Institute for Qualitative Methodology. 11(1): 13–25.

Sweet, L. (2002). Telephone Interviewing: Is It Compatible with Interpretive Phenomenological Research? Contemporary Nurse: A Journal for the Australian Nursing Profession. 12(1): 58–63.

van Manen, M. (2006). Writing Qualitatively, or the Demands of Writing. Qualitative Health Research. 16: 713. DOI: 10.1177/1049732306286911

Varga, S. (2001). Authenticity as an Ethical Ideal. New York: Routledge.

# 12 Inseeing to the heart of the matter

*Kent Smith*

## Abstract

The purpose of this chapter is to explore my lived experiences of becoming and being a hermeneutic phenomenological researcher. The story that follows is "my style" that emerged by doing, and so my contention is that each experience of hermeneutic phenomenological research is a unique lived experience. This acknowledges, there are shared universalities that may be attuned to and so offer an experience of research that is intuitive and revealing. Although not a methodological way of researching, it is a way of bringing understanding to researchable questions related to lived experience. What you will read in this chapter is how I came to understand that dwelling in the tension of using phenomenological writing is a way to reveal notions meaningful to the research question and through example show how the core notion revealed in my research, that of inseeing, surfaced. Finally, I share what was revealed to me as implicit to Being-a-hermeneutic-phenomenological-researcher.

## My practice of phenomenological research

Imagine an emerging philosopher at his desk gazing into the vast expanse of his mind. What is he seeing "in there"? For sure, he is in there seeing something. That something is an experience of coming towards the thing, what thing? It is a tension; he is not yet sure what this thing is. He suspects he will know, but at this point, he does not. He is building something, though, building a Becoming experience. He knows it will arrive – he's whistling a tune from the new Dylan album – he loves that song "I Contain Multitudes." Building, building, building! Outside of him family, observe him at the writing place and ask:

> What's he building in there?
> He's hiding himself from the rest of us
> He's all to himself, I think I know why
> And what's that tune he's always whistling?
> What's he building in there?
> We have a right to know.
>
> (Waits 1999)

DOI: 10.4324/9781003081661-12

This chapter explores some aspects of my journey of building and revealing my way of Being-a-hermeneutic-phenomenological-researcher and how this emerged from within myself.[1] Those that observed this process in action were very curious as to the building of the research methodology and many questions ensued. I come from a family of researchers – and none familiar with hermeneutical phenomenology. In particular, my chapter will wonder about how the notion of "inseeing" opened interpretive possibilities for my researcher self. Looking back to my building a research way, I now see that I was always a Becoming-phenomenologist – I just didn't know it!

Engaging in a hermeneutic-phenomenological research project necessitates Becoming a hermeneutic-phenomenological person. Becoming is within Being.[2] I noticed this experiential shift about midway through a doctoral study, and in the noticing was that this way of researching and Being profoundly changed both the research and myself as a researcher. It felt like a slow quiet metamorphosis, and I didn't at first notice it, writing in my study. Rather I first noticed the shift in my day job – that of doing counselling. I, in my counselling practice, was always Becoming-a-phenomenologist. Of course, this is the way it is – seeing the world through who and how I am, "*from one way of being to another 'in the twinkling of an eye'*" (Groth 2001, 82). In counselling, I was starting to look into the meaning of the client's experiences and moving away from counselling technique and symptom focus. I also noticed how I always wrote as an act of counselling practice. Reflexively there was an awareness of a shift in this process of how I "do" counselling writing and this writing started to resemble phenomenological writing.

Looking back at the counselling writing shift, and also into two academic research projects (Smith 2006; 2018), I see how this shift "in the twinkling of an eye" occurred through the lived experiences of Being-a-counsellor and the connected living experiences of Being-a-researcher. This connection was the transitional awareness of "twinkling" moments being connected and so altered the way I encountered researching thereafter. I recall my supervisors being very happy with this shift. It was an important moment for me as a researcher because up until then, I was attempting to research as I had previously counselled – with a technique and strategy orientation. I noticed in my master's thesis (Smith 2006) that when commenting on research methodology, my position as the researcher was to "*develop an appropriate methodology of research that was meaningful for counsellors*" (6). Where I looked for this was to the social sciences, where "*counsellor researchers typically pull their methodologies from social science theories*" (6). There was not a mention of ontology when I wrote that thesis chapter. Conversely, the methodology chapter in my doctoral thesis started with ontology and this shift in understanding between the two thesis methodology chapters is extraordinary to me in reflection. Ontology, I noted, as the study of Being itself is "*the only worthy subject of a phenomenological philosophy*" (Speigelberg 1994, 352). Three new words in my research vocabulary – ontology and phenomenology and philosophy. New and familiar.

The choice of phenomenology as a research methodology was clear to me. Not only was this approach the congruent methodology for my research subject, but congruent with me as a researcher and being a counsellor! Being a counsellor led me to this genre of researching as my counselling work revealed notions of Being that demanded to be explored. My doctoral research project explored the not yet revealed phenomenon of Becoming-a-counsellor-leader. Being leaderful was the thing that the research eventually opened up into a notion in and of itself. Looking back, I chose hermeneutic phenomenology as a philosophic structure to frame the way to research. Yet it is also clear now there was no other way. Looking back often clarifies because it reveals that hermeneutic phenomenology chose me.

As a counsellor I am an existential therapist. I had worked with many clients with what Cohn (2002) proffered is "'The Rule of Description', [which] is summed up as 'Describe, don't explain' – explanation is seen as a limitation. It has no place in Heidegger's hermeneutics ..., which knows no final answers" (73). This phenomenological way of counselling was what was familiar as I grappled with researching – and with that "twinkling," there was my already known inspiration for counselling and the previously hidden and newly uncovered inspiration for researching:

> What is it that phenomenology is to 'let us see'? ... What is it that by its very essence is necessarily to the theme whenever we exhibit something explicitly? Manifestly it is something that for the most part does not show itself at all: it is something that lies hidden ... but at the same time is something that belongs to what thus shows itself, and it belongs to it so essentially as to constitute its meaning and its ground. Yet that which remains hidden in an egregious sense, or which relapses and gets covered up again, or which shows itself only 'in disguise', is not just this entity or that, but rather the Being of entities.
>
> (Heidegger cited in Cohn 2002, 74)

In the hiddenness and the not showing, Heidegger describes that meaning is often in murky dark places and at the same time, is often hiding in the light and in plain sight. Heidegger (1962) went on to write about the importance of the priority of the phenomena:

> This Being can be covered up so extensively that it becomes forgotten and no question arises about it or about its meaning. Thus, that which demands that it becomes a phenomenon, and which demands this in a distinctive sense and in terms of its ownmost content as a thing, is what phenomenology has taken into its grasp. (59)

Heidegger's study of the phenomenon is familiar through existential counselling theories. This familiarity was hidden to me, it was at the same time known and unknown. When reflecting on my researcher-Being, the familiarity became "seen." It was the twinkle twinkling, it was wondrous in its wonder, it was an essential moment that shifted my understanding, suddenly it was seen – voilā there it is! From the counselling theory books (Cohn 2002; LeBon 2001; Spinelli 2001; van Duerzen-Smith 1997; among many other others) to Being and Time (1962) – there was a connection. This beautiful connection is where hermeneutic phenomenological research and counselling together demand that what lies hidden is uncovered, shows itself as it is, and so meaningful possibilities emerge. Suddenly I was a hermeneutic phenomenologist. A counsellor-researcher-philosopher-counsellor. In this emergence, a phenomenon became distinctive and grasped and the notion of inseeing as an aspect of a Becoming-a-researcher showed itself.

This notion of inseeing appears out of the depths of Heidegger's (1962) Being and Time and shone a light on what could be – it was an "a-ha" moment for me. Possibilities illuminated and I felt free to live within the space Heidegger described as the "*tension of emerging and not emerging*" (Petzet 1993, 143). In this tension, I was whistling a tune that became very familiar and welcomed a notion that chose itself to be the centrepiece of my research. This is an interesting phenomenon in itself – the notions reveal themselves and the researcher must be attentive to their appearance. I certainly found that this was now me; attuned and open-to-Being-researcher.

## Tension of emerging and not emerging

Being-a-researcher means simultaneously loving and fearing the tension of emerging and not emerging possibilities. As the wonderful lyricist Patterson Hood sings, "there's a voice within the void, and I swear it sounds familiar" (2020). This familiar voice is within the stories of the people who engage with the research. The familiar voice is also within the stories of the researcher, and so when the researcher and the people connect, something new unfolds. This is the place of emergence, and as a hermeneutic phenomenologist, this is where the tension resides. What will come from this? Is it of value? Will it be of interest? What is it?

I recall speaking with a fellow researcher who, at the time, was four years into his Ph.D. write-up. He had chosen hermeneutical phenomenology as his methodology and talked about the void. The emergent was not emerging – he was frightened. Choosing hermeneutical phenomenology can be an act of courage. The search is to see the essence of the experience in the stories once collected and contend with the anxiety of needing to develop the consistent story of sorts and to keep grounded in the "*lived experiences [that] are the data of phenomenological research*" (van Manen 2017, 814). van Manen (1997) articulates that the role of the researcher is to bring "*into nearness that which tends to be obscure*" (32). This is no easy task. Indeed, when I start interpretation, it always requires some courage to take interpretive leaps to find and see the obscure.

In my doctoral thesis (Smith 2018), I wrote my way as the following:

> I read the participants' responses as written transcripts of taped interviews in full many times and I wondered about and noted down tentative essential themes at each reading. I read the scripts aloud to myself, and I listened.

Sometimes I noticed something that I had not seen whilst only reading. It was related to mood, my mood of being pulled into the content. (105)

Mood or attunement is an aspect of Becoming for me. What I mean by this is in entering the research itself, I became a philosopher. This, in my experience, is a necessary condition towards interpreting. In ordinary moods (those of not being a philosopher), my courage is not there nor is my noticing of the emergent – I'm not *in*. The tension in not being there leaves me barren. Being-in the philosopher mood connects to the felt experience of researching:

It was about noticing something that 'felt' important to the story of the study. Inspiration was a distinct mood that came from the stories of the participants. Sometimes the inspiration was the simpleness of the everydayness of the lived experience of ordinariness. Sometimes it was inspiration as experienced by the extraordinary experiences shared. I noticed, that although hard to find a way in, once in I was pulled into the whole of the combined stories.

(Smith 2018, 105)

"*In*" is the mood that I attuned to in engaging – it made me courageous. My *in* mood enables everydayness to become visible as a something wondrous. *In* is living in the tension of emerging and not emerging. *In* is connecting to the whole in such a way that philosophic meanings open up where they had not before. *In* is my experiencing the space between a priori and a posteriori: the place between knowledge before knowledge and knowledge as experience lived. In my thesis, I describe how *in* gets connected to seeing:

I reflect that is the challenge: where to enter the hermeneutic circle. Certainly, once entered, one is in the centrifugal flow of part and whole (Gadamer 2013). I found that when in this flow, phenomenological 'inseeing' occurred (van Manen 2017). van Manen (2017) articulates 'inseeing' as a glimpse into the hidden nature or a view beneath the surface. (105)

Inseeing in this sense evokes meaning insights. Meaning insights are different from general insights, meaning insights come from wonder, the mood that transports us "*in*" to "*the beginning of genuine thinking*" (Heidegger cited in van Manen 2014, 37). Genuine thinking is that that leads to wonder, a mood that is deep and reveals phenomena "*saturated with meaning*" (van Manen 2014, 37). The mood of wonder is different in the research mood, it is felt; and so, courage, inspiration and wonder are all embodied so as to be "in." What is being described here is the mood of Becoming-a-researcher. That is, the mood leading into interpreting and ongoingly re-interpreting data, which reveal an embodied standpoint (Spinelli & Marshall 2001). van Manen (2017) explores this:

Meaning insights tend to occur when we wonder about the sense or the significance of the originary of an experiential phenomenon. Originary does not mean new or original. Originary means inceptual: originary insights reveal the primal meaning and significance of a phenomenon. (822–823)

Originary is not original, originary is inceptual; inceptual through the engagement of the lived experience. In my experience of being phenomenological these beginnings are a result of Becoming-a-philosopher. This notion might seem an unusual description of the notions we are investigating in these chapters – how to be a hermeneutic phenomenological researcher. Nevertheless, it is my experience of embodiment. In order to do hermeneutic phenomenological research, one must be *in* the ongoing always experience of Becoming-philosopher. *In* there lies the gaze of inseeing – beautifully described by Rilke:

> If I were to tell you where my greatest feeling, my universal feeling, the bliss of my earthly existence has been, I would have to confess: It has always, here and there, been in this kind of in-seeing, in the indescribably swift, deep, timeless moments of this divine seeing into the heart of things.
>
> (cited in van Manen 2017, 68)

I wonder if this divine experience of inseeing is what Heidegger (1966) was considering in his dwelling on meditative thinking? He described meditative thinking as "*thinking which contemplates the meaning which reigns in everything that is*" (46). Meditative thinking, he considered, is a way of thinking we have lost because we have become too absorbed in technology and the fast-paced world (van Duerzen-Smith 1997). So, we have therefore lost aspects of what thinking is and can be. Inseeing takes me back to this meditative thinking experience. Indescribably swift, deep into an embodied experience of the heart of things. This may sound like a mystical experience in its description – nonetheless, it is a research experience to savour and love.

Researching this way is a mystical experience of reading, speaking, listening, reflecting, and seeing the whole giving a glimpse into a broader history of lived experience in order to consider where originary meaning insights emerge. Back to the story of my thesis experience:

> There was a sense of knowing that as essential themes emerged to me that there would be connection to philosophy. Trusting that I could follow the flow of inspiration from what I already knew into what I did not know was a process of interpretive understanding. At this time, I began referencing back to the Heideggerian notions that held a strong and orientated relationship with the essence of the stories. Going back to reading returned me to notions of phenomenology to more fully consider the inspiring themes selectively and separately from the whole script and brought me back to the philosophy. This process of "reading and re-reading deepened the essence of the stories, not always clearly, and sometimes as 'revelatory.'"
>
> (Smith 2018, 106)

Apparent in this description is the importance of immersing oneself in the research material in order to assimilate as much of the *"explicit and implicit meaning as possible"* (McLeod 2003, 85). Added to these experiences of Becoming I found my phenomenological self in the art of writing and re-writing. This is where much of the immersion took place and where the emergent emerges. These were revelatory moments which I will never forget and where, in writing, I found a new space in which to "see-in."

## The art of writing and re-writing is inseeing in-action

Writing in and out, all over the place, around and around, the stories of self, the stories of others, the stories, the stories – to the stories themselves – there it was! Writing is a way of immersion and the *"act of writing itself forms the research process of ... hermeneutic phenomenology"* (Cohen, Kahn, & Steeves 2000, 74). Writing is a vital research method in that it is a *"way of finding out about yourself and your topic"* (Richardson 1994, 516). Historically, I write because I want to understand something and develop my ideas. This is the opposite to the experience of writing when I know something and have something to say (Richardson 1994). Writing for the purpose of research begins for me in the form of a reflexive research journal. This reflexive journal included notes on methodology, observations, conversations and anything else pertinent to the research and specifically develops into a book of meanings (Richardson 1994). This helped me maintain a strong and orientated relationship with the study (van Manen 1997). By the time of interpretation, the writing and re-writing had provided a connection to interpretive depth and formed a crucial aspect in the *"movement from identification and comparison of themes to a coherent picture of the whole"* (Cohen, Kahn, & Steeves 2000, 81). Indeed, writing as a style of interpretation is a *"way of 'knowing' – a method of discovery and analysis. By writing in different ways, we discover new aspects of our topic and our relationship to it"* (Richardson 1994, 516).

Phenomenology is philosophical researching and researching is writing and in writing the researcher is a writer. To quote van Manen (2014), *"one finds it impossible to write. And yet one must write. One is drawn to write. One writes. One has become 'one' who writes"* (359). This is, in my experience, the tension of emerging and not emerging. In becoming one who writes, the phenomenological writer attunes to this tension. In being attuned, and in maintaining a strong and orientated relation to research writing, space opens up in text that provokes insights that are *"more real than real"* (362). This is the interpretive stance where revelations occur (Gadamer 2013). My writing moments are experiences of externalising meanings, delivered from inside to the world, as Sartre (1939) suggests:

> everything is finally outside: everything, even ourselves. Outside, in the world, among others. It is not in some hiding-place that we will discover

ourselves; it is on the road, in the town, in the midst of the crowd, a thing among things, a human among humans. (2)

This type of writing opens the ability to "see," see things I could not *see* previously in the felt meaning of the story (van Manen 1997). Inseeing can elicit essences that are uncovered from the layers of language that have covered the phenomenon. The text of the phenomenological researcher, therefore, succeeds only when it lets be seen *"that which shines through, that which tends to hide itself"* (van Manen 1997, 130).

I still try to recollect the experience as it was. Luckily, I have my writing to remind me – and I am feeling something here and now too that makes the re-member of my Becoming-a-researcher clearer. Writing this chapter is taking me back and I re-member writing about writing:

> It is in the process of writing that I find my connection to the parts and the whole of the story of the research. One is a phenomenological writer. Of course, one is always becoming a writer. The journey is fraught. When a segment of a research's script was considered as a story that could be used to develop the argument threaded through my research story, I carefully craft in order to create flow, without losing the participant's voice. Adams and van Manen (2017) articulate that this is the "rhythm of "anecdote/reflection" … [where] the anecdote/reflection pair consists of a carefully crafted lived experience description, followed closely by a reflection on an aspect or aspects of the phenomenon given in the anecdote." (788)

This process opens textual tone and aspect seeing (van Manen 2014). To articulate the notions of textual tone and aspect seeing in a text van Manen (2014) wrote that when "inseeing" into the text, what we find *"is less the outward particularities than the dawning experience of recognition that the external appearance makes possible"* (263–264). Seeing-in is a view that offers possibilities. These possibilities are the exciting emergent experiences of research projects. Coming to the experience of writing as open-to-Being, the words of the writing twinkled here and there – like the stars on a clearing night.

In considering aspect seeing,[3] van Manen (2014) acknowledges Heidegger: *"Aspect names and also is that which constitutes the essence in the audible, the tasteable, the tactile, in everything that is in any way accessible"* (cited in van Manen 2014, 263). The point here is that written text speaks and in so doing can uncover philosophical notions if it is listened to and/or read intensely enabling the *"task of letting us "see" this implicative meaning in an explicative manner"* (van Manen 2014, 264). The experience described by van Manen offers research as an artistic endeavour, one where the linguistic freedoms of philosophy and literature can create an evocative depth of beauty in the interpretation and writing. Phenomenological researching allows stories to flourish and grow into a wide-ranging exploration of the emergent. Writing as a phenomenologist prompts *"our mode of attending and perceiving [which] has the effect of sculpting different domains or territories of experiencing"* (Pearmain 2001, 69). The phenomenological mode as described here is in honour of the phenomenological imperative: to describe life as we live it.

> I – nurture the one track taking flight
> Let it surround me like a starry night
> Let it hypnotize, puncturing the minds.
> (Crutchfield 2020)

Writing phenomenologically metaphor and description reveal the mysterious into a notion, *"making it new, and giving it back almost unchanged except in that it had been observed"* (Bakewell 2016, 237). Of course, what is observed can be seen as so ordinary that it cannot be the thing itself until it is. In my doctoral research, the thing itself, Being-leaderful, was a gift from a participant, yet it seemed so ordinary in the conversation and in the reading, it was looked past so many times. I recall not being able to see-in until many writing and re-writings had occurred – and the emergent slowly emerged – there it was – the thing itself – the notion of my research emerged. Writing, in my experience, is the tension between the emerging and not emerging.

## Seeing-in or inseeing

Let's go back to Heidegger's (1962) thoughts on "seeing." He writes that the *"seeing of 'ideas' is the primordial kind of uncovering"* (26). As I understand this, Heidegger is acknowledging that seeing ideas is an experience of Becoming. It is a *"way of Being-in-the-world, [that] the most primordial 'truth' is the 'locus' of assertion; it is the ontological condition for possibility that assertions ... may uncover or cover things up"* (269). Heidegger is directing us to the importance of the Being-thereness of temporal awareness where *"care is grounded [in] the full disclosedness of the 'there'"* (402). Only in this the space of Being-thereness is there possibility for *"clearedness [toward] any illuminating or illuming, any awareness, 'seeing', or having of something, made possible ... for its existential possibility"* (402). Heidegger is leading us into the radical ontology of phenomenology (Crotty 1998). In this radical place, notions such as inseeing are enlivened and enlightened in such a way to enable the Becoming-a-researcher to reach the place where contending with the anxiety of being is an absolute necessity. Seeing the twinkling in the experience of Becoming-a-phenomenological-researcher requires a climb into dizzying heights of unknownness for the uncovering to emerge. Heidegger describes an ontological seeing as the:

> remarkable priority of 'seeing' ... for we do not say 'Hear how it glows', or 'Smell how it glistens', or 'Taste how it shines', or 'Feel how it flashes'; but we say of each, 'See'; we say that all this is seen ... We not only say, 'See how that shines', when the eyes alone can perceive it; but we even say, 'See how

that sounds', 'See how that is scented', 'See how that tastes', 'See how hard that is.' (1962, 215)

The revelation of "seeing" uncovers possibilities for the openness-of-Being. Heidegger (1962) refers to "seeing" as a way of "*Being … that … shows itself in the pure perception which belongs to beholding, and only by such seeing does Being get discovered. Primordial and genuine truth lies in pure beholding*" (215). This is the experience that oscillates between literal-perceptual sight: indeed, it is the experience of moving and flowing between metaphorical-historical "seeing" and literal-perceptual "seeing." Lakoff and Johnson (1980) consider stories as ideas that reveal and light up, and that discourse is the medium towards the "seeing." They explain that through the dialogue of the story openness-of-Being is revealed:

I see what you're saying. It looks different from my point of view. What is your outlook on that? I view it differently. Now I've got the whole picture. Let me point something out to you. That's an insightful idea. That was a brilliant remark. It really shed light on the subject. It was an illuminating remark. The argument is clear. It was a murky discussion. Could you elucidate your remarks? It's a transparent argument. The discussion was opaque. (470)

Meaningful insights are phenomenological in-seeings (van Manen 2014; 2017). van Manen (2014) writes this is getting to the "*sheer pleasure of insight and feeling touched by things that reach the depth of our existence and confirm our humanness*" (68). In-seeing brings an understanding of how lived experiences have and do reveal the meaningfulness of current living experiences.

## Trouble with classicists

The trouble with a classicist he looks at a tree
That's all he sees he paints a tree
The trouble with a classicist, he looks at the sky
He doesn't ask why, he just paints sky
(Lou Reed & John Cale 1990)

Phenomenologists see the tree physically and describe it as it is. Phenomenologists also get as close to the tree in order to see the tree, and then within the description, we become mystified with the non-physical:

mystified by the commonplace, [we] move effortlessly, into the strange, until nakedness frightens, confounds, and he seeks a bit of cover, order. He glimpses, he gleans; piecing together a crazy quilt … the cruel intensity of this process can produce a thing of beauty but oftentimes just a tear in the shimmering from which to wrest and wiggle. A spine of rope sliding an arena more remote and dazzling than ever.

(Smith 2011, 13)

Possibilities are drawn from the experience wrest and wiggling, finding the twinkling and dazzling, yet remote until it is close. Then we "see", both physically and non-physically, as Wittgenstein reflected, "*I suddenly 'see' the presence of something*" (cited in van Manen 2014, 264). In my experience, this is where inseeing insights occur. In this texture, an emergence. Seeing the emergent, one way or another, as an ambiguous dawning of presence (van Manen 2014).

## Clearing

Writing is a flow that variously gets stuck. In these moments, one is in the tension – the emergent, not yet emerging. Knausgaard (2016) describes the writer's need for mood as he explores the colour of the writing mood:

> there was no such colour in what I wrote, no such hypnotic or evocative mood, in fact there was no mood at all, and that is the heart of the problem, I assumed, the very reason I wrote so badly … The question was whether I could acquire such a colour or mood. Whether I could fight my way there or whether it was something you either had or you didn't have. (159)

Part of my process is to find the spaciousness to create flow. I noticed the more stuck I become the more I need to find my way out of my way as that "*which is un-ready-to-hand in this way is disturbing to us*" (Heidegger 1962, 103). In other words, when not able to see the wood for the trees, I feel there is no path. To find my path and reduce disturbance, I surf, and this is how I described the experience of surfing as a research experience to my doctoral supervisor:

> I get really angsty when there isn't any swell. If there's swell you're always torn to go 'oh'. But there's none so just write. But sometimes I've just gone out and paddled out and just sat out there anyway. Absolutely thinking really, because there's nothing else to do there. It's a wonderful experience. It's the experience of the lapping of the little wave, of the little swell on the board. And something just moves up the body through that core, that emotional place where sometimes you feel that emotion. You know people talk about the hairs on the back of your neck or something. You sit there and it just comes. And then always and without exception, and this is an absolute for me, I'll go back, and I'll be able to just write probably for the rest of the afternoon without really even stopping to think. That's my clearing.

In this clearing, clearedness occurs, an experience where there is space to dwell and uncover, conscious or unconscious uncovering layers of meaning. Dahlstrom describes Heidegger's clearing notion this way; "*the clearing is the 'free region' where other things are present, coming across or standing opposite one-another … the 'openness' … affords any possible appearing or showing*" (2013, 45). The free region, the clearing is going back to the experience of Being. For me, this is often around disputing the learned experience for the lived experience. What I mean by this is that we often go into institutions or enter academia to learn and reflect on theory, however, when we enter the so-called real world, we do the real thing. For me, this is weaving surfing into my research experiences and my life experiences. Surfing brings me into nearness allowing the reverberation of meaning to become attentively recognised (van Manen 2014). Heidegger (1962) describes his notion of clearing,

> To say that it is 'illuminated' ["erleuchtet"] means that as Being-in-the-world it is cleared [gelichtet] in itself, not through any other entity, but in such a way that it is itself the clearing. (171)

What is useful to note here is that the illumination is not a light switched on out there in the world; rather, Dasein switches on a light for him/herself, in the doing, in his/her interaction with the world. Generally, the world is categorised and created for the workman in the context of his particular concerns: he sees a missed deadline in a half-finished [ridden] barrel (Royle 2018).

I, the researcher, am a workman tools down, riding the barrel. My surfing clearing reminds me I have it – the writing mood. Writing mood is as my surfing mood – *in* – into the heart of things. I found after a surf and in front of the screen and with renewed energy the emergent emerges, "*Only for an entity which is existentially cleared in this way does that which is present-at-hand4 become accessible in the light or hidden in the dark*" (Heidegger 1962, 171). The following is an example of the actual experience where the light was shone on the notion that eventually was the core of my doctoral thesis. Here follows a lived experience description of a Becoming moment for a research participant:

> I think I've always been somewhat leaderful in the way I approach the world. So, as I'm the eldest daughter, I'm also the eldest grandchild of my generation, and I think I've always taken up that position in a way that just said, 'I get to have opinions, or bring something to that'. I think my father was very much, you're the eldest, you're responsible, your sisters follow you, you have to set a good example. (*Kathryn*)

So, what did I do with this story? The following is part of my interpretive write up of this story:

> Leaderful is a wonderful description of an 'approach to the world' of a leader. Kathryn is bringing attention to the aspect of self (and family positionality) as she in reflection, brings life to herself as a leader, as a person who leads. She describes her leaderful self as being built on her confidence of considerable inner resources that enable the sense of engaging in the world optimistically. Although prior to any thought of being in a leading role, this reflection of

a lived experience highlights her sense of being able to engage with a challenge, that is full of possible anxiety, and find a sense of personal strength and self-advocacy.

(Smith 2018, 130)

It was a moment after surfing, deeply into my thesis dwelling that I *see* the *leaderful* notion uncovered. Heidegger (1962) leads me to the thought that in surfing, there is the project of removing that which is disturbing me and thus *"enables us to see … that with which we must concern ourselves in the first instance"* (103). With the disturbance quelled, he writes, in this *"looking around,"* the referential context of Being is *"lit up"* (105). By the opening of the space of the missing disturbance, it is as if a light switches on and the world that has always existed has been there all along, now *"announces itself"* (105) and is revealed.

> I take no action and the people are transformed themselves;
> I prefer stillness and the people are rectified of themselves;
> I am not meddlesome and the people prosper of themselves;
> I am free from desire and the people of themselves become simple
> like the uncarved block.
> (Tao Te Ching, as cited in Dryden & Mytton 1999, 57)

As I sit here writing, I am actively re-membering these experiences, which are experiences of the continuances of Becoming-a-researcher. Of course, we never "are," ongoingly the Becoming evolves and so this writing experience today enables a mood of lit up. Again, Heidegger (1962) is helpful to the experiences of writing about the beforehand experiences of writing *"The environment announces itself afresh. What is lit up is not itself just one thing ready-to-hand"*[5] (105). It is the continuous nature of Being-a-person. It reminds me that Becoming-a-researcher is an ongoing experience of being alive.

## Being-a-researcher is Being-alive

Becoming-a-phenomenological-researcher opened the world for me personally. The experiences, particularly in the interview conversations and the writing, illuminated my – me. I was captivated in staring out the window for long periods of time – dwelling into the stories of participants in my study. When the twinkling started and the stories lit up, tension subsided and meaning insights emerged. Often, I was stunned by what emerged – indeed, I still wonder! Nevertheless, although there is no specific method to hermeneutical phenomenology research, there is a way. I hope this chapter of my experiences shows this. Again, looking back, I wrote in my thesis experience the following:

> Throughout this study I have been very aware of time: time as a linear concept and time as in 'this doctoral journey is a great time in my life'. Coming to this reflection I am aware that time is moving on and an end

is coming. I have become very conscious of the influence of this research process on my own counsellor-leader presence. Of particular interest to me is how research has added so much to my counselling practice. I acknowledge that the stories of the counsellor-leaders of this study have been especially influential in this. I felt, during this study, fulfilled by my counselling community and colleagues. Research has brought me back to 'the thing itself'. That 'thing' for me is the exploration, through being a counsellor-leader, of social change.

(Smith 2018, 214)

These thoughts of the-then-researcher have remained strong for the now-counsellor-leader. What has happened for me is that the experience of research has taken me time and time again back into the stories of the study. Although there is no product as an outcome of my doctoral thesis, there is ongoing living of it. "That everything returns" is indeed as Nietzsche observed. *"the closest [possible] approximation of a world of Becoming to a world of Being"* (Arendt 1971, 18). It is as Heidegger (1962) pointed to that my researcher-Being has *"been laid open"* (105). In being laid open, my world has expanded and research itself has altered the very course of my life – on a day-to-day basis. This is no small admission; the course of my life has changed every day as a lived and living experience. There are other ways to conduct research, however, in my "now" lived experience, it is unlikely that there would be as personal an outcome in other approaches that I am describing here. This is not the researcher immersing himself into the research, rather the research immersing the researcher. Again, to Heidegger (1962);

> when something ready-to-hand is found missing, though its everyday presence [Zugegensein] has been so obvious that we have never taken any notice of it, this makes a break in those referential contexts which circumspections discovers. Our circumspection comes up against emptiness, and now sees for the first time what the missing article was ready-at-hand with, and what it was ready-to-hand for. The environment announces itself afresh. (105)

It all comes together and when it does the environment announces itself afresh. Inseeing the very presence and recognition of the present-at-hand, the that which is already there, then we are invited to play a part (Bergson 1994). It sure did happen that way for me!

## What it means

What has happened in writing this chapter has replicated my doctoral research. I have gone backwards into lived experiences to insee the meaning inceptual in Becoming-a-phenomenologist. That is, a philosopher who thinks meditatively and poetically about the things themselves and interprets. Becoming a researcher then, I reminded myself, was always going to be Becoming-a phenomenologist!

What it means to be a phenomenologist is to be courageous. There is no straight-ahead playbook (although I found van Manen 1997; 2014 very helpful). A phenomenologist must set their own course. If one is open to this, the journey is nothing less than exciting.

> I was feeling sensations in no dictionary
> He was less than a breath of shimmer and smoke
> The life in his fingers unwound my existence
> Dead to the world alive I awoke
>
> (Smith 1996)

When one exits the study, one may be profoundly altered and so the road in is a different one than the road out the other side. Personally, this is a good reason to take the risk with this research way. However, one must be courageous and be prepared for an existential experience – at times crisis and at times seeing into the heart of things like never before.

> Writing shows that we can now see something and at the same time shows the limits or boundaries of our sightedness. In writing the author puts in symbolic for what he or she is capable of seeing. And so, practice, in the lifeworld …, can never be the same again. My writing as a practice prepared me for an insightful praxis in the lifeworld. (I can now see things I could not before.) Although I may try to close my eyes, to ignore what I have seen, in some ways my existence is now mediated by my knowledge.
>
> (van Manen 2014, 130)

As you have read these pages on hermeneutic phenomenological research, it will be clear that the research way is philosophic. In my mind, the world currently needs more philosophers engaging in the modern world questions. There is much already known as well as wisdom in our collective histories that is available to be mined and used to consider what it is to be alive. If you head into research with a hermeneutic phenomenological gaze, firstly make sure you have an excellent supervisor and then be open to the following:

> Research is a piece of art – be creative.
> Love the tension and fear the tension.
> Trust there is a process of phenomenology, which you will create.
> The lived experience of the researcher is a resource that must be mined.
> Seeing in and out; what is inseen must become outside.
> Heidegger is tough to understand – find sources who have already done the hard work.
> Heidegger is magnificent once understood – it's worth the work.
> Stare out the window – a lot.
> See the twinkles twinkling and luxuriate in those moments of emergence.
> Surf

# Notes

1. Parts of this chapter are drawn from my notes and writings in my doctoral thesis. The thesis research was granted ethical approval by the Auckland University of Technology Ethics Committee on 26th August 2015 (Smith 2018).
2. By Becoming and Being, I am utilising Richardson's interpretation of Heidegger's meaning of Being, that is "that man is not a being like other beings but enjoys a prerogative all his own by reason of which his own Being is not from the beginning a *fait accompli* but something that he himself must achieve" (2003, 28).
3. Aspect seeing is explored in detail by van Manen (2014, 264).
4. The clearing provides accessibility to that that is available. Then that is present-at-hand can be seen and so used. Present-at-hand is a term Heidegger used to differentiate Being from world, from this point of view present-at-hand is *reality* (1962, 228).
5. In becoming afresh, Heidegger is pointing to the fact that the ready-to-hand is "'there' before anyone has observed or ascertained it" (1962, 105).

# References

Adams, C. and M. van Manen. 2017. "Teaching phenomenological research and writing." Qualitative Health Research, 27 no. 6: 780–791. http://dx.doi.org/10.1177/1049732317698960

Arendt, H. 1971. The Life of the Mind: The Groundbreaking Investigation on How We Think. New York: Houghton Mifflin Harcourt Publishing Company.

Bakewell, S. 2016. At the Existentialist Café: Freedom, Being, & Apricot Cocktails. London: Vintage.

Bergson, H. 1994. Matter and Memory. Translated by N.M. Paul and W.S. Palmer. New York: Zone Books.

Cohen, M.Z., D. Kahn, and R. Steeves. 2000. Hermeneutic Phenomenological Research: A Practical Guide for Nurse Researchers. London: Sage Publications, Inc.

Cohn, H. 2002. Heidegger and the Roots of Existential Therapy. London: Continuum.

Crotty, M. 1998. The Foundations of Social Research: Meaning and Perspective in the Research Process. Crows Nest: Allen & Unwin.

Crutchfield, K. 2020. Hell. On Saint Cloud [Recorded by Waxahatchee]. Tornillo: Merge Records.

Dahlstrom, D. 2013. The Heidegger Dictionary. London: Bloomsbury Academic.

Dryden, W. and J. Mytton. 1999. Four Approaches to Counselling and Psychotherapy. London: Routledge.

Gadamer, H.-G. 2013. Truth and Method. Translated by J. Weinsheimer and D. Marshall. London: Bloomsbury Academic.

Groth, M. 2001. "The body I am: Lived body and existential change." In Embodied Theories, edited by E. Spinelli and S. Marshall, 81–97. London: Continuum.

Heidegger, M. 1962. Being and Time. Translated by J. Macquarrie and E. Robinson. Oxford: Blackwell Publishing.

Heidegger, M. 1966. Discourse on Thinking. Translated by J.M. Anderson and E.H. Freund. New York: Harper and Row.

Hood, P. 2020. Awaiting Resurrection. On The Unravelling. Memphis: ATO Records.

Knausgaard, Karl Ove. 2014. Boyhood Island: My Struggle Book 3. Translated by D. Bartlett. London: Vintage.

Knausgaard, K.O. 2016. Some Rain Must Fall: My Struggle Book 5. Translated by D. Bartlett. London: Vintage.

Lakoff, G. and M. Johnson. 1980. "Conceptual metaphor in everyday language." The Journal of Philosophy, 77 no. 8: 453–486. Retrieved from https://library.aut.ac.nz/

LeBon, T. 2001. Wise Therapy. London: Continuum.

McLeod, J. 2003. An Introduction to Counselling (3rd ed.). Buckingham: Open University Press.

Pearmain, R. 2001. The Heart of Listening: Attentional Qualities in Psychotherapy. London: Continuum.

Petzet, H.W. 1993. Encounters and Dialogues with Martin Heidegger, 1929–1976. Translated by P. Emad and K. Maly. Chicago: The University of Chicago Press.

Reed, L. and J. Cale. 1990. Trouble with Classicists. On Songs for Drella – A Fiction. Sigma Sounds. New York: Sire Records.

Richardson, L. 1994. Writing – A Method of Inquiry. Handbook of Qualitative Research, edited by N. Denzin and Y. Lincoln, 516–529. Thousand Oaks, CA: Sage Publications, Inc.

Richardson, W. 2003. Heidegger: Through Phenomenology to Thought (4th ed.). New York: Fordham University Press.

Royle, A. 2018. "Heidegger's Ways of Being." Accessed 12 September 2018. https://philosophynow.org/issues/125/Heideggers_Ways_of_Being

Sartre, J.-P. 1939. "Intentionality: A Fundamental Idea of Husserl's Phenomenology." Accessed 22 March 2019. https://www.stephenhicks.org/wp-content/uploads/2016/05/Sartre-JP-Husserl-Intentionality.pdf

Smith, K. 2006. "In the Room: The Question of Counsellor Presence." MA Thesis, Victoria University of Wellington.

Smith, K. 2018. "Out of the Room: A Phenomenological Study into the Lived Experiences of Becoming and Being a Counsellor-Leader." DHSc Thesis, Auckland University of Technology.

Smith, P. 1996. Dead to the World. On Gone Again. Electric Lady. New York: Arista Records.

Smith, P. 2011. Woolgathering. London: Bloomsbury Publishing.

Speigelberg, H. 1994. The Phenomenological Movement: A Historical Introduction (3rd ed.). Dordrecht: Kluwer Academic Publishers.

Spinelli, E. and S. Marshall. 2001. Embodied Theories. London: Continuum.

van Duerzen-Smith, E. 1997. Everyday Mysteries: Existential Dimensions of Psychotherapy. London: Routledge.

van Manen, M. 1997. Researching Lived Experience: Human Science for an Action Sensitive Pedagogy. Toronto: Best Book Manufacturers.

van Manen, M. 2014. Phenomenology of Practice: Meaning-Giving Methods in Phenomenological Research and Writing. Walnut Creek: Left Coast Press.

van Manen, M. 2017. "Phenomenology in its original sense." Qualitative Health Research, 27 no. 6: 810–825. http://dx.doi.org/10.177/1049732317699381

Waits, T. 1999. What's He Building? On Mule Variations. Cotati: Anti.

# 13 Attuning to trustworthiness and final reflections

*Gill Thomson and Susan Crowther*

## Abstract

In this final chapter, we focus on how to achieve trustworthiness in hermeneutic phenomenology (HP) studies and offer some final reflections for those embarking on or using HP in their work. Trustworthiness and rigour are central concepts to achieving quality in research – they encompass whether the design and methods are appropriate and an assessment of the quality, authenticity, and veracity of the research. Trustworthiness and rigour tend to be used interchangeably in the wider literature, though trustworthiness is generally perceived to be more aligned with qualitative methodologies. Here, we draw on the etymological meanings of these terms and question whether either is suitable for the unbounded nature of HP studies.

While there are different frameworks and criteria for "trustworthiness" in existence, here we use the work of Lincoln and Guba's due to their broad and encompassing concepts. We use their framework to re-visit the work of the chapter authors; the concepts of credibility, confirmability, dependability, transferability, and reflexivity are used as a lens to consider how quality in HP studies can be achieved. Each chapter has shown how HP is able to be sculpted by the researcher's focus on a lived experience and phenomenon of interest by attuning in a certain way and adopting a phenomenological attitude. We contend that while HP is a creative, and flexible methodology, a similar style can be adopted when attuning to "quality." Accommodating methods can be used while not compromising a methodology that strives for "showing" ontological depths. In the final sections, we offer closing sentiments about how the use of HP can be perceived as political. HP offers a differing perspective to the "gold standards" of positivist methodologies super-valued within the research community. The HP approach can be perceived as a less privileged methodology due to not operating within a rigid methodological and easily replicable framework. HP studies are also often limited to postgraduate dissertations due to difficulties in obtaining funding. We close by offering some final sentiments as to where next in the use of HP and the challenges and gifts of using this approach.

## What is in a name?

Determining the components and criteria for rigor in qualitative research has and continues to be hotly debated (Morse 2015). Rigor and trustworthiness are used interchangeably in the literature to describe the process of assessing the quality of qualitative-based research (and evident amongst our chapter authors,

DOI: 10.4324/9781003081661-13

for example, Chapters 3 and 4). In line with a Heideggerian approach, it is important to consider the etymological meanings of these words (an approach also used by Margot in Chapter 8). The term "rigour" stems from Old French and Latin words such as "strength," "hardness," "firmness," "be stiff" and "exactness, strictness without indulgence." Whereas trustworthiness (or trust) stems from old Norse and Proto-Germanic terms such as "faithfulness," "confidence," "trust," "fidelity," "be firm, solid steadfast" and "that on which relies" (etymology. online). It is easy to reject rigour being assigned to qualitative research due to all its terms depicting a fixed and exact approach that points to a specific "truth." Trustworthiness (or trust) includes some terms aligned with qualitative methodologies, such as "confidence" and "faithfulness" – but others describe an immutable truth and a need for rigid (solid) and predefined, exact (fidelity) methods. These definitions mean that rigour and trustworthiness are either completely or partially antithetical to a HP study. While challenging to try and introduce new terms in an area that (albeit superficially) is "understood" by the wider academic audience, and perhaps beyond what we achieve here, we contend that a search for a new language is needed. We consider that terms such as "integrity" defined as the quality of being honest, the state of being whole and undivided (from Old French terms such as soundness, wholeness, correctness), or "credibility" (from Medieval Latin "quality of being credible, capacity or condition of being believed") may be more suitable.

We continue to use the term "trustworthiness" here in recognition of our shared understanding. But, like Heidegger, rather than continuing to use terms handed down that are welded with positivistic notions of validity, certainty and replication, this debate should continue.

## What do we mean by quality?

It is argued that quality standards are needed to provide an authoritative evaluation of "good" research:

> The worth of any research endeavour lies in the hands of the researcher(s) and their ability to demonstrate rigour and auditability.
>
> (Carter 2006, 55)

Historically, however, it has been a challenge for interpretive scholars to adopt a methodological framework that is situated within its philosophical roots and one which demonstrates academic rigour through a trustworthy and dependable analysis. This is largely due to the available frameworks being developed for positivistic sciences where the focus is on objective controls, adherence to predefined criteria, and on replicability.

In a qualitative study, it is impossible to apply the same rigor and control. For this reason, assessing quality in qualitative research has been a well-debated topic, and only recently has there been *any* consensus on what constitutes a "good" qualitative study (Hadi and Closs 2016). Rolfe (2006) details three opinions on how to judge qualitative research. The first, least popular opinion advocates for assessments of validity and reliability to be used in qualitative research. The second, challenges the value of a single pre-determined criterion for evaluating the quality of diverse qualitative approaches. This is of particular relevance to HP work due to its flexible, unbounded approach meaning that no standardised "measure" is possible or even desired. The third, and in our opinion, the most suitable (also referred to as the "realist" methods), promotes criteria more aligned with the ethos and value of qualitative research (Rolfe 2006); where criteria offer flexibility so that the different methods align with the theoretical and methodological approach adopted.

Porter (2007) provides a useful argument towards different approaches to "validate" qualitative research. He argues against views of qualitative research being judged by readers on its aesthetic criteria and believes that each methodology needs its own approach. He considers that if qualitative research is to provide a viable alternative, then there needs to be some quality assessment undertaken, and that "realist methods" *"holds out greatest promise"* (Porter 2007, 79). We agree with this position. If we want our work to be taken seriously and as a wise colleague – Professor Liz Smythe – once told me, there has to be a "so what" to our work. Participants gift us rich in-depth insights often on an altruistic basis to improve the situation of others. Flexible, and creative criteria that enables us to do this in a way that demonstrates "quality," has to be a good thing. When using HP in applied research, we surely do not want this to be a purely academic endeavour; rather, for our work to be read as a credible source of evidence that can raise awareness, educate, inform, challenge mindsets, and make a difference. To achieve this, we need "some" adherence to quality standards.

There are different criteria to assess "quality" in qualitative research. For example, de Witt and Ploeg (2006) describe concepts such as "balanced integration" – concerned with congruence between the philosophical underpinnings of the study, the topic of the research and the researcher. "Openness" relates to providing a detailed audit trail. "Concreteness" aligns with reflexivity in regard to presenting researcher pre-understandings in order to be *concretely in the context of this phenomenon*" (225). Concreteness also refers to usefulness of the study, the "so what." "Resonance" – the "phenomenological nod" – the gesture of agreeing, the unspoken nod of resonance and mutual understanding from the reader (also see Liz and Deb, Chapter 2). Finally, "actualisation" relates to what is produced – for example, a peer-review journal, presenting at a conference, informing a practice-based guideline, advising on policy or educational curriculum relates to "actualising the study." In the following sections, we use the four interlinking criteria described by Lincoln and Guba (1985) and draw on examples from the chapter authors and wider literature to describe how the quality of HP studies should be undertaken. We use Lincoln and Guba's (1985) criteria over others due to familiarity; because their concepts are inclusive and encapsulate essential elements of quality that align with qualitative research; and their work tends to be the most well used.[1] In the following sections, we describe Lincoln and Guba's four criteria – "credibility," "dependability," "confirmability" and "transferability" – and re-visit the work of our chapter authors to offer examples of how each can be achieved. We also consider reflexivity. While this is not directly referred to in the work of Lincoln and Guba, it is an inherent element of "confirmability." Reflexivity is fundamental to HP studies and thus discussed throughout by our chapter authors. Nonetheless, to not address here as a central tenant of "trustworthiness" would be amiss.

## Credibility

Credibility relates to whether the research findings represent a credible conceptual interpretation of the participants' original data (Lincoln and Guba 1985). It aligns with de Witt and Ploeg's notion of resonance and the "phenomenological nod." Credibility is achieved when research

> ... presents descriptions of interpretations of human experience that others having that experience would immediately recognise.
>
> (Lincoln and Guba 1985, 296)

Smythe et al.'s (2008) view considers that an untrustworthy HP study would be one that "tells" rather than shows the reader (4). Credibility, therefore, encompasses how HP studies are written; HP studies need to present ontological understandings that invites the reader to "think-along" with a shared resonance. An invitation to think along attunes the reader to the unconcealing nature of phenomenological prose drawing the readers of our work into the adventure of encountering differing horizons of understandings guiding them into a fusion of horizons in the showing.

A personal moment of credibility in my (Gill) Ph.D. was when I presented my interpretations to some of my research participants. My PhD was a HP study of psychological birth trauma. A number of the women from my study had joined a theatre group to act out scenarios of their personal birth experiences in professional forums; the intention being to raise awareness and to enact positive change. An unplanned situation occurred when I and the theatre group were presenting at the same conference. It was suggested by my primary supervisor that I should offer a private presentation for my participants. I can still recall feeling completely overwhelmed at the suggestion – what if I caused distress – what if they didn't like how I had interpreted their stories – what would this mean for my study? During the presentation, I could see some of them crying; afterwards they told me how they had felt "*heard*." For one woman, listening back to the stories enabled her to recognise why she had been "*stuck*" on her traumatic birth (rather than her other experiences of childbirth). For Susan, sharing crafted stories with a woman who had experienced a challenging homebirth that resulted in an instrumental birth in the local hospital provided credibility in her study. The woman reported how beautiful it was to be reminded and "see" the beauty, joy and celebration that the birth had been for her and everyone there sharing the event; reading her own story was a healing and remembrance of specialness. Polly (Chapter 3) also describes how she witnessed a *"stillness"* in the audience when presenting her poems at a medical conference and how afterwards a doctor told her he was now going to change his practice to hear the voices of children/young people in his care. Credibility occurs when others connect with what is shared; with Kvale and Brinkman (2009) identifying how the retelling of the stories has the potential to improve the human situation. This was certainly the case in our experiences.

Credibility or the "phenomenological nod" (Smythe 2011) can also be sought when discussing findings with work colleagues and peers or presenting the work at events and conferences. This is a process also referred to as "peer debriefing" (Holloway and Wheeler 1996), or "analytic triangulation" (Hadi and Closs 2016). It can involve conversations about the research methodology, data analysis and interpretations continuously throughout the research process. Josh (Chapter 10) referred to these opportunities as a "playful debate" that enabled his pre-understandings to be challenged. Everyday conversations with those outside of the participant group can also allow the surfacing of further insights (Smythe et al. 2008). For Margot (Chapter 8) and for participants in Liz and Deb's study (Chapter 2), belonging to a Heidegger reading group helped to facilitate sense-making of Heideggerian notions and what was surfacing in their data.

Another strategy to improve credibility, and similar to the definition provided above, relates to "prolonged engagement" (Lincoln and Guba 1985). Prolonged engagement concerns an investment of sufficient time in the research to become oriented to the phenomenon of interest. The purpose is to render the inquirer open to multiple influences and interpretations (Lincoln and Guba 1985). This approach concerns immersion in the collected stories, in-depth engagement and use of philosophy and wider theoretical insights to underpin the study's epistemological, ontological, theoretical, methodological and interpretive approach. HP is a study of thinking, thinking, and more thinking. As the chapter authors highlight, they thought about the stories and wider readings *everywhere*, while out walking (Polly, Chapter 3), surfing (Kent, Chapter 12), on a treadmill (Helen, Chapter 7). For Margot (Chapter 8), and others, this process also involves connections to wider resources such as novels, films and poetry. HP researchers need to be openly engaged in searching everywhere to find insights that can help unconceal meanings for ontological depth.

A further method to enhance the credibility of the findings refers to "member checking." Member checking is a rather contested area due to challenges of "checking" on a situated conversation that transcends the researcher and the researched. Sandelowski (1993) challenged the need for member checking as stories constantly change due to ongoing temporal changeable nature of personal and social agendas. Morse (2015) also argues against opportunities for participants to change their minds – an approach not required in other types of research. A long time ago, I (Gill) was asked by the project lead to return transcripts to participants to "check." On reflection, a rather ill-informed idea, as at that point, no analysis had been undertaken, and therefore uncertain as to what was being "checked." I only had two responses, both to tell me how unpleasant they had found reading their verbal prose. In my Ph.D. of birth trauma, I did what I called a "final interpretation" meeting; this involved re-visiting all the participants to share early thoughts and interpretations of their stories. While appreciably less congruent with HP due to the temporal nature of our understandings, I stand by it as an approach aligned with credibility. This meeting invoked acknowledgements and invited further depths to their experiences. It offered another level of immersion, and as aligned with Heidegger's philosophies, it opened up a shared clearing of understanding, and through which further meaning was generated. The approach I used shares similarities with Bridget's (Chapter 4) work, whereby she used the second interview as an opportunity to reflect on insights shared during the first interview. Helen and Elizabeth (Chapter 7) also detail a collaborative shared interpretive approach between the researcher and participant, and in situations when this could not be achieved real-time, the interpretations were sent separately for feedback and comments.

Furthermore, while not credited as "member checking" per se, a method gaining ground in HP studies is through returning crafted stories (Crowther et al. 2017) to participants (and an approach employed by a number of the chapter authors, such as, Christine's work in Chapter 9). This process is meant to be less about member checking than to bring forth agreement about felt meanings (Zambas and Wright 2016). The participants in Susan's Ph.D. provided appreciative feedback to how the returned stories *"had crystallized their meanings."* Polly Livermore (Chapter 3) also discusses the positive feedback she received from the two participants to whom she sent their crafted poems. On an ethical and practical level, sending crafted stories to participants also provides an opportunity for them to ask for sections and/or whole stories to be redacted. For example, in a study by Susan on the lived experiences of remote-rural midwives participants requested specifics removed because of fears of reprisals and censure if they were identified due to the small population working in these regions.

## Dependability

Dependability emphasises the need for the researcher to account for the ever-changing context of the research and is responsible for articulating the integrated processes of data collection, data analysis, and theory generation. One of the ways this criterion can be achieved is through some form of auditable process. Lincoln and Guba (1985) consider that comprehensive methodological documentation is essential. A key point of criticism by John Paley (amongst others) relates to how meaning is generated in phenomenological-based research – one of his latest texts (Paley 2016) draws on published examples to discredit HP as well as other phenomenological approaches. His focus is on exposing how the interpretations are based on the researcher's prior inferences; whereby a biased gaze is used to confirm pre-suppositions rather than uncover hidden meanings. Thus, the key challenge to achieve auditability in HP studies is for the reader to follow the HP writer's decision-making and associate it with their own conclusions drawn from the information provided.

Dependability encompasses all methodological details such as recruitment sources and techniques, data collection and analysis (Hadi and Closs 2016). This is also referred to as providing "thick descriptions" (Long and Johnson 2000) that requires providing sufficient methodological and analytical details. Arguably, some of this information is easier to detail than others. While the emphasis of our book was to highlight *how* we make the interpretive leap – the tension is making it explicit *exactly* what occurred during this process is still evident. Some of the chapter authors refer to *aha* moments of generating understanding (such as described by Polly in Chapter 3 when crafting her first poem), or the use of in-seeing (Kent, Chapter 12), or keeping *"swimming"* (Christine, Chapter 9) whereby meanings would be revealed. Whereas others offer more detailed insights into the methodological processes followed (for example, see Polly, Chapter 3, Bridget, Chapter 4 and Lesley Kay, Chapter 5). HP authors have different styles, and we contend these should be honoured. Dependability for HP studies is not about a prosaic linear formula – but it does need to show readers how you came to point to that particular phenomenon. A reflexive diary plays a central role in reporting all aspects about the study such as documenting significant changes about the methodological and theoretical design of the research. It is also used to explicate all the initial and progressive thoughts, ideas, and meanings as the interpretive work progresses. A number of our authors such as Polly (Chapter 3), Christine (Chapter 9) and Jean (Chapter 11), stress the importance of having a notebook or journal on hand at all times to capture the thoughts and insights – the signs and pointers to what is calling in the data – that emerge through dreams, on the bus, out walking, in unrelated conversations and so on. All of which is an important detail for dependability.

A key goal of HP research is to "show" the reader how the interpretations were always-already-there, waiting to be uncovered; our aim is to point to what was hidden from view and to invite them to think. It requires good use of participant data and a seemingly effortless blend of philosophical and theoretical insights, so the links between them is obvious. This book is populated with rich examples of how this can be achieved, such as Bridget's (Chapter 4) use of Heidegger's views of technology and parts and pieces to illuminate how sexuality and intimacy is experienced when living with a life-limiting illness, and Christine's (Chapter 9) insightful and varied examples of Heidegger's notion of *care* in the everyday world of being-alongside in Human Resource Management.

## Confirmability (and reflexivity)

A further method identified by Lincoln and Guba (1985) is "confirmability" – the degree to which the findings are the product of the focus of the inquiry and not the biases of the researcher. This criterion has evident similarities with credibility and the phenomenological nod and with dependability in terms of the reader being "shown" how the interpretations are grounded in the data. However, a key feature of confirmability, while not emphasised by Lincoln and Guba, relates to reflexivity.

Positivist methodologies utilise fixed pre-defined schedules to collect what they consider to be objective data, unbiased by researcher input. Whereas interpretive-based qualitative approaches such as HP recognise and value that we cannot "bracket" our inherent, unconscious, and pre-reflective ways of knowing (also see Chapter 1); a situation perceived as impossible by Heidegger, Gadamer and others since. HP researchers, and as reflected by all chapter authors, acknowledge our end result as being a "fusion" of horizons of philosophical underpinnings, the participant data, wider readings and our pre-understandings. However, employing caution not to settle on superficial and sentimental understandings is crucial. A key premise of reflexivity is to protect again what Heidegger refers to as "vicious circle;" whereby we interpret based on what we knew already.

Researchers gravitate towards HP studies because of their own personal and/ or professional experiences with the phenomenon of interest. For me (Gill), my motivation to undertake a doctoral study of birth trauma was fuelled by my own personal experience of a negative and difficult birth, for Susan, the Ph.D. journey begun with a feeling of loss and perceived covered-up-ness of something special at birth in a biomedically informed 21st-century childbirth dominated culture after 30 years in midwifery practice. For Polly (Chapter 3), it was her experience of caring for young people with Juvenile Dermatomyositis, for Lesley Kay (Chapter 5), her impetus to study birth stories was based on her experiences as a mother and as a midwife, whereas for Lesley Dibley (Chapter 6), her attraction to researching a stigmatised group (those living with inflammatory bowel disease) called to her due to her identity as a gay woman. It is rare, in our opinion, to meet researchers who use this approach who have no experientially infused (vicarious or otherwise) stimulus. Why this passion drives and stimulates us to HP projects, it also holds potential dangers of our fore-structures of understanding influencing what we hear and interpret in our data. Our fore-conception, a sense of what our interpretations will be is perceived to the *"most dangerous aspect of understanding"* (Smythe and Spence 2012, 16). This danger stems from Heidegger's notion of the *"The They"* (also see Chapters 5 and 11) whereby we interpret based on the everyday understandings handed down to us by those in our social worlds, and where *Dasein's* understanding is lost and covered over.

A common reflexive technique (also see Liz and Deb Chapter 2, Polly Chapter 3, Lesley Kay Chapter 5, Kent Chapter 12, amongst others) is to be interviewed at the start of the research process. This provides an invaluable opportunity to reflect on why we are undertaking the study and, more importantly, an opportunity to identify our conscious and unconscious pre-understandings. With this in mind, it is crucial to think about who best to be the interviewer. Both Susan and I have offered this to our own and other students who we meet on our HP course. Whoever you select, they need to have an understanding as to what we mean by reflexivity and its essential nature in informing a HP project. I (Gill) and Jean (Chapter 11) also wrote our own birth stories at the beginning of our studies to help unpack and reflect on our pre-reflective ways of knowing. This information (interview, stories) then becomes the start of our reflexive diary. The intention of the interview, writing personal accounts and the reflexive diary is not to set our pre-understandings aside while we look anew, but rather, as called for by van Manen (1997), to engage in an openness that reveals our orientation and attunement to the phenomenon. An example is provided by Lesley Dibley (Chapter 6) whereby she reflects on how she (and her family) adapted their personal situation to prevent being "Othered," and which in turn helped her to further understand her participant's experiences. Christine (Chapter 9) also considers how reading and re-reading her own stories of *care* as a daughter, mother, employee and manager helped to provide a renewed perspective in understanding the meanings of others. Pre-understandings need to be made explicit and to be explored and challenged to avoid biased subjectivity (Kvale and Brinkman 2009). Highlighting our pre-understandings throughout serves to mitigate this and opens our inquiry to scrutiny.

Peer debriefing (as discussed above) helps to safeguard against "vicious" interpretations, such as through regular discussions with supervisory, peers or wider research teams to discuss decision-making and interpretations generated. Time to read and re-reflect on each interview, and before undertaking the next, is also important to consider how certain questions invoke certain responses, and what further questioning or prompts could be used. As Josh reflects (Chapter 10), taking time, particularly after the initial interviews enabled him to question his interviewing approach, and the need to adjust his approach to capture stories rather than purely theoretical reflections. In my (Gill) Ph.D., sharing early transcripts with my supervisors helped me to see how my perception of trauma was influencing what prompts I asked and what I was hearing. Furthermore, the experience shared by Lesley Dibley (Chapter 6) about her interviewing approach offers a useful example of how we need to start within, so we can become attuned to the voices of others. Oftentimes new HP researchers focus on "doing" their interviews and "getting them done" without taking the time to dwell with each interview. Susan often asks postgraduate students to "slow down and savour" – this is thoughtful contemplative research, not hasty procedural research. Although not always feasible to do 1–2 interviews per month, due to logistics of recruitment, travel costs and organisation of the interviews, our advice would be not to hurry the data collection. Taking the time and being-with each interview brings unexpected insights (for example, about yourself, the data, the context) that may be obscured by overloading oneself with multiple interview data all at once.

## Transferability

The final technique to achieve trustworthiness relates to "transferability." This represents the extent to which the findings resonate to wider contexts outside of the study situation (Lincoln and Guba 1985; Sandelowski 1986). This criterion differs to generalisability – a hallmark of quality associated with quantitative-based studies. Generalisability is when research findings based on a population sample are applied to the population at large. Transferability, while similar in terms of its aim in making wider inferences, does not involve broad claims and rather invites the reader to make the connections.

Transferability is believed to be accomplished when findings are well-grounded in life experiences and reflect typical and atypical elements (Sandelowski 1986). It also concerns providing detailed information about who the participants are and potential factors that may help to make sense of the interpretations generated. It calls for detail on the wider political, cultural, and social context in which the stories were captured. This is not as a means of causality but to situate their lived experience as part of a nuanced, context-related *Being-in-the-world*. Jean (Chapter 11), for example, highlights the wider tension the midwives faced when introducing homeopathy within their midwifery practice. Polly (Chapter 3) links the child/young person's age to the crafted poems. Bridget (Chapter 4) links the interpretations to the participant's different life limiting condition to aid understanding. While Lesley Dibley (Chapter 6) also considers wider sociocultural influences in helping to understand the stigma that participant's experience from family and others in relation to their inflammatory bowel disease. HP studies never claim for generalisable truths, but equally, one of its characteristic features is to instil a sense of knowing and resonance in others; knowing where and how the stories were captured and with whom aids this process.

## Final reflections

In our final reflections, we explore how HP is political and where HP as a research method is travelling. In one of our previous publications, we argue how phenomenology is political, situated within wider debates of how research agendas (such as RCTs, process evaluations) can exert power to achieve dominion over the "interpretive qualitative-based methodologies" (Crowther and Thomson 2020). The dominant discourse in research continues to be that experimental-based studies are the gold standard to evidence-based care. However, quantitative data alone is privative in helping to reveal human experience. Qualitative research is increasingly used alongside trial designs in order for studies to not only answer questions as to whether a particular intervention "works" or not (via quantitative-based responses) but also use of qualitative insights into why it worked for whom, when, etc. Such an approach arguably enables more rich and comprehensive insights to inform future intervention design. HP studies, on the other hand, offer something distinct. It is not an appropriate approach to use in assessing a specific intervention, but rather it aims to honour the interconnected relational totality of a particular lived experience. It aims to look beyond the everydayness and surface the pre-reflective meanings to understand the "is-ness" of what it "is." Alongside qualitative studies (for example, mixed methods approaches) generally aim for explanation, causation, and theory-building. Conversely, HP offers a powerful means to "see" into the world of others and to generate experiential, situated implications.

A key way in which we observe the dominion of positivistic methodologies relates to the lack of funding for HP studies; it is almost exclusively relegated as a methodology for post-graduate HP studies. We have consistently witnessed how HP is underfunded and resource poor (Crowther and Thomson 2020). The sample size in HP research is inevitably small and debated by a number of our chapter authors (see Jean in Chapter 11 and Bridget in Chapter 4). Bridget, for example, includes a large sample due to the felt pressure of a larger sample holding more weight in a research community that super-values quantity over quality. Though, important to note in her reflections that were she to start again, she would not have taken this stance. To do HP well, means that dwelling, and thinking on the data needs time; it calls us to attune differently to a mood of wonder and openness. The data that HP research generates directs our reading in a myriad of journeys – when I (Gill) heard the "heroic" qualities in my work, I searched databases, the internet, read fiction and poetry to help me understand the heroic elements that were always-already there, but not yet spoken. If this process is curtailed too soon, there is a danger of the interpretations being superficial and descriptive. As HP interviews explore lived accounts of a particular experience that has relevance and meaning for the individual, this inevitably creates a voluminous amount of text. As suggested previously, take the time to dwell with each interview. Even small numbers of interviewees generate an extensive amount of information that needs careful attention and attunement. Unfortunately, this is an approach less valued in an academic community that super-values generalisability and proof. Our position, however, is that HP studies need to be a standalone endeavour, or, as a minimum, an arm of a mixed-methods study with sufficient resources and time available to honour what is required. How the meaning focused findings of HP analysis can navigate vastly different epistemologies and ontologies and be appropriately incorporated and equally valued in a mixed methods study is the subject for a further article or/and chapter.

Despite the increase in use and value of qualitative research such as being integrated with quantitative evidence to inform clinical and international guidelines (World Health Organization 2018), we are definitely not there in valuing the gifts of HP endeavours. We, and as detailed by a number of our chapter authors, have encountered continuing challenges, inequalities, and inequities. For example, challenges within research careers (where the push is to become more aligned with wider research methodologies that generate funding and successful grant capture), editorial and reviewer preferences (publications and conferences), and formulaic ethics applications. A Ph.D. student at one of our HP courses told us how he had to make numerous revisions to his ethics applications due to wanting to capture lived accounts of children in a relatively innocuous subject area – their experiences of outdoor education. Conveying "trustworthiness" in HP projects in published articles is also highly challenging due to wordage constraints. Restricted word lengths can make it impossible to convey all the iterative and in-depth processes involved in HP work. We also face problems when trying to publish our work with editors and reviewers aligned with positivistic approaches and undervaluing the ideographic and emic accounts of participants. When I (Gill) was trying to publish my first study from my Ph.D. I entered into a battle with one reviewer. This individual was trying to insist that I made reference to women's experiences being based on unrealistic experiences rather than situating their experience within an individual-social-health service *Being-in-the-world* perspective. The compromise was for me to emphasise that it was the women's subjective accounts that I was reporting. One of Susan's first HP publications met challenges due to the style of mantic and pathic writing, an emotive feeling quality in academic prose that comes with a sense of prophetic significance[2], a style that bubbles up when writing hermeneutically. Eventually, after some correspondence, the editor told Susan that she enjoyed the quality of writing and acknowledged that as an editor she had been resistant to that genre of reporting. Bridget (Chapter 4) also reports on numerous challenges she has experienced when publishing such as reviewers disputing the use of first person, being asked to provide a rationale for not using multiple-rater agreement in the generated interpretations, having to justify not using a structured and replicable interview schedule and an expectation of returning interpretations to participants for validation purposes. All situations aligned with a positivistic frame of reference.

There are numerous new directions for how HP work is evolving and developing. The work of Helen and Elizabeth (Chapter 7) demonstrates how HP can be developed by drawing on the work of Merleau-Ponty and others to create an embodied HP approach. Polly's (Chapter 3) work also describes how a range of creative approaches were used to "hear" the voices of those often marginalised from research – children and young people. There have also been moves in using HP data in different and powerful ways. Body maps (see Chapters 3 and 7), diary methodologies, observations, and photo-elicitation to accompany in-depth phenomenological-based interviews also offer exciting directions to use multiple ways of seeing and hearing lived accounts. There are always new ways in which the data and interpretations generated by HP studies are being used. For example, Jenny Patterson et al. (2019) used her HP findings to inform a filmed expressive dance that depicts the discord in providing woman-centred maternity care. Steph Heys (one of Gill's Ph.D. students) captured vulnerable/disadvantaged women's lived accounts of maternity care to inform a script; the script was then filmed using a 360-degree perspective to be replayed using Virtual Reality headsets. Wright-St Clair et al. (2011) photographed the hands of the elderly undertaking their favourite activity in an occupational therapy HP study revealing the phenomenon of being aged. All these examples have produced visual methods designed to be used within health professional forums to invoke emotion and action. They demonstrate how HP through its capacity to capture rich, powerful, lived accounts can be used for political gains to raise awareness and reconnect healthcare providers to human aspects of caring.

As referred to at numerous points throughout this book, HP is not "one" thing. Unlike an RCT with fixed, immutable protocols, with "any" deviations perceived as a breach, it is a fluid, flexible approach that is ever-evolving while still staying "true" to its fundamental and essential underpinnings. HP studies need to draw on the work of Heidegger, Gadamer, and others to inform the methodological, theoretical, and interpretive decisions and to use open-ended approaches to capture the lived reality of "Being there." HP prioritises reflexivity and philosophy; this is its strength (in terms of the depth of meaning that can be generated), and also its weakness (due to it being perceived as overtly subjective) (Crowther and Thomson 2020; Paley 2016). HP as a research method faces political and methodological challenges about what research is and is not. Rather than merely perceiving attacks such as the work of John Paley as mere criticisms, we need to see these as a call to action and to show what HP is capable of. We need to demonstrate congruence and to be complicit with "trustworthy," for want of a better expression, practices. Our work (for example, Crowther 2019; Crowther and Thomson 2020; Thomson et al. 2012), this book, as well as the work of others, for example, the recent book by Dibley et al. (2020) and Josh Spiers' (2019) monograph are dedicated to this cause. We invite you to continue this plight.

The power of HP is its ontological uncovering; when done well, we do not have had to have experienced the phenomenon, yet we can "come to feel" what it is like through the evocative rich interpretations created. However, as alluded to throughout this collection of works, HP is not an easy task. We need to *become* phenomenological, and for those of us less used to such a philosophical approach, it can seem an impossible task, particularly when engaging in the dense and impenetrable readings of Heidegger. The challenge, as articulated by Christine and Kent (see Chapters 9 and 12), is to have courage and trust. Courage to keep going, and trust that in time the understanding and meanings will come. As Josh advises (Chapter 10), start with the work of others (that is, Blattner 2006; Dreyfus 1991; Harman 2006) who can provide us with a basis of understanding to then engage in Heidegger's work direct. There is never going to be a quick win to "find" "phenomenon" in HP work. While we consider, as discussed earlier, that the term "trustworthiness" may not be entirely fit for purpose, it does hold important connotations of trust. Trust that we will find the way to uncover what the phenomenon *is* – trust to listen, to think, to ponder, to ask some more, and to wait for the glimpses and qualities to call forth.

HP studies need time and patience to do it well, and we need to attune to the space where we can be free from other noises, such as ontic concerns or the voices of The They; to let go, to dance to the sound of what we hear, and to enter into the clearing when a mood of wonder can be invoked and embraced. We need time to read and re-read the transcripts or other data generated, to follow what calls out in the data back into philosophical and theoretical texts, and to reflect on our own pre-understanding, all of which will point to what was there, waiting to be uncovered. It requires what is referred to as existential dwelling (see Margot, Chapter 8) or genuine, meditative thinking (see Kent, Chapter 12), to find meaning, see the obscure and to touch the primordial. All our authors described feeling unsettled, anxious, uncertain, overwhelmed and frightened of not finding their way and for the phenomenon to be forever hidden from view. Equally, they all refer to how exhilarating and enriching HP is. It is a journey of wonderment and awe that touches us in such unexpected ways as we become transformed through Heideggerian thinking, and when we intuitively "know" and "see" what was *always-already* there, while being mindful that we are never truly "done" and there can always be more to see. At times it can feel like traversing the unknown in a tempest, yet yielding to the process can say "it" so much better when we decide to let go and to leap in. Mary Oliver says this so eloquently in her poem "The Storm":

> Now through the white orchard my little dog
> romps, breaking the new snow
> with wild feet.

> Running here running there, excited,
> hardly able to stop, he leaps, he spins
> until the white snow is written upon
> in large, exuberant letters,
> a long sentence, expressing
> the pleasures of the body in this world.
> Oh, I could not have said it better
> myself.[3]

We believe, as all of our chapter authors, that we don't find HP, rather HP finds us, and by reading this book, you are already on the path – so take heart, engage in *"the gift of the struggle"* (Smythe and Spence 2019, 7) and leap into the "white orchard" expressing your delight as you further reveal what it means to be alive.

## Notes

1. This is not to imply that other criteria used are 'wrong' or 'insufficient'. What is meant here is that the criteria discussed are, in many ways, overarching concepts that resonate with other suggested criteria such de Witt, L. and J. Ploeg (2006).
2. For more on mantic writing in HP studies, see van Manen, M. 2014. *Phenomenology of Practice: Meaning-Giving Methods in Phenomenological Research and Writing*. Left Coast Press.
3. Mary Oliver's "The Storm" – 2017, 31: Devotions – The selected poems of Mary Oliver, Penguin Press, New York; The poem is originally from Dog stories 2013.

## References

Blattner, W. 2006. *Being and Time: A Reader's Guide*. London: Continuum.

Carter, B. 2006. "'One Expertise among Many' – Working Appreciatively to Make Miracles Instead of Finding Problems: Using Appreciative Inquiry as a Way of Reframing Research." *Journal of Research in Nursing* 11 (1): 48–63.

Crowther, S. 2019. *Joy at Birth: An Interpretive, Hermeneutic, Phenomenological Inquiry.* London: Routledge.

Crowther, S., Ironside, P., Spence, D. and Smythe, E. 2017. "Crafting Stories in Hermeneutic Phenomenology Research: A Methodological Device." *Qualitative Health Research* 27 (6): 826–835.

Crowther, S. and Thomson, G. 2020. "From Description to Interpretive Leap: Using Philosophical Notions to Unpack and Surface Meaning in Hermeneutic Phenomenology Research." *International Journal of Qualitative Methods* 19. doi: 1609406920969264

de Witt, L. and Ploeg J. 2006. "Critical Appraisal of Rigour in Interpretive Phenomenological Nursing Research." *Journal of Advanced Nursing* 55 (2): 215–229.

Dibley, L., Dickerson, S. Duffy, M. and Vandermause, R. 2020 *Doing Hermeneutic Phenomenological Research: A Practical Guide*. London: Sage.

Dreyfus, H.L. 1991. *Being-in-the-World: A Commentary on Heidegger's Being and Time, Division I*. Cambridge, MA: MIT Press.

Hadi, M.A. and Closs, S.J. 2016. "Ensuring Rigour and Trustworthiness of Qualitative Research in Clinical Pharmacy." *International Journal of Clinical Pharmacy* 38 (3): 641–646.

Harman, G. (2006). *Heidegger Explained: From Phenomenon to Thing*. Chicago, IL: Open Court Publishing Company.

Holloway, I. and Wheeler, S. 1996. *Qualitative Research for Nurses*. Oxford: Wiley-Blackwell.

Kvale, S. and Brinkman, S. 2009. *Interviews: Learning the Craft of Qualitative Research Interviewing*. Los Angeles: Sage Publications.

Lincoln, Y. and Guba, E.G. 1985. *Naturalistic Inquiry*. Thousand Oaks, California: Sage.

Long, T. and Johnson, M. 2000. "Rigour, Reliability and Validity in Qualitative Research." *Clinical Effectiveness in Nursing* 4 (1): 30–37.

Morse, J.M. 2015. "Critical Analysis of Strategies for Determining Rigor in Qualitative Inquiry." *Qualitative Health Research* 25 (9): 1212–22.

Paley, J. 2016. *Phenomenology as Qualitative Research: A Critical Analysis of Meaning Attribution*. London: Routledge.

Patterson, J., Hollins Martin, C.J. and Karatzias, R. 2019 "Disempowered Midwives and Traumatised Women: Exploring the Parallel Processes of Care Provider Interaction That Contribute to Women Developing Post Traumatic Stress Disorder (PTSD) Post Childbirth." *Midwifery* 76: 21–35.

Porter, S. 2007. "Validity, Trustworthiness and Rigour: Reasserting Realism in Qualitative Research." *Journal of Advanced Nursing* 60 (1): 79–86.

Rolfe, G. 2006. "Validity, Trustworthiness and Rigour: Quality and the Idea of Qualitative Research." *Journal of Advanced Nursing* 53 (3): 304–310.

Sandelowski, M. 1986. "The Problem of Rigor in Qualitative Research." *Advances in Nursing Science* 8 (3): 27–37.

Sandelowski, M. 1993. "Rigor or Rigor Mortis: The Problem of Rigor in Qualitative Research." *Advances in Nursing Science* 16 (2): 1–8.

Smythe, E. (2011). "From Beginning to End: How to Do Hermeneutic Interpretive Phenomenology." In G. Thomson, F. Dykes, and S. Downe (Eds.), *Qualitative Research in Midwifery and Childbirth: Phenomenological Approaches* (pp. 35–54). London: Routledge.

Smythe, E., Ironside, P., Sims, S.L., Swenson, M. and Spence, D.G. 2008. "Doing Heideggerian Hermeneutic Research: A Discussion Paper." *International Journal of Nursing Studies* 45 (9): 1389–1397.

Smythe, E., and Spence, D. 2012. Re-viewing literature in hermeneutic research. *International Journal of Qualitative Methods* 11(1): 12–25.

Smythe, E., and Spence, D. 2011. "Reading Heidegger." *Nursing Philosophy* 21 (2): e12271.

Spier, J. 2019. "Authentic Caring: An Australian Experience." In *Strategies for Facilitating Inclusive Campuses in Higher Education: International Perspectives on Equity and Inclusion*. Bingley UK: Emerald Publishing Limited.

Thomson, G., Dykes, F. and Downe, S. 2012 *Qualitative Research in Midwifery and Childbirth: Phenomenological Approaches*. London: Routledge.

van Manen, M. 1997. "From Meaning to Method." *Qualitative Health Research* 7 (3): 345–369.

World Health Organization. 2018. *WHO Recommendations on Intrapartum Care for a Positive Childbirth Experience*. World Health Organization. https://www.who.int/publications/i/item/9789241550215

Wright-St Clair, V.A., Kerse, N. and Smythe, E. 2011. "Doing Everyday Occupations Both Conceals and Reveals the Phenomenon of Being Aged." *Australian Occupational Therapy Journal* 58 (2): 88–94.

Zambas, S.I. and Wright, J. 2016. "Impact of Colonialism on Māori and Aboriginal Healthcare Access: A Discussion Paper." *Contemporary Nurse* 52 (4): 398–409.

# Index

Printed in the United States
by Baker & Taylor Publisher Services